Neurobiological Foundations for EMDR Practice

Uri Bergmann, PhD, is in full-time private practice, in Commack and Bellmore, New York. He is an EMDR Institute Senior Facilitator and Specialty Presenter as well as an EMDR International Association Approved Trainer and Consultant in EMDR. He is a lecturer and consultant on EMDR, the neurobiology of EMDR and the integration of EMDR with psychodynamic and ego-state treatment. Dr. Bergmann has authored and published articles on the neurobiology of EMDR in peer-reviewed journals and has contributed chapters to various books on EMDR. He is a member of several journal editorial boards.

Dr. Bergmann is a past-president of the EMDR International Association (EMDRIA) and is currently serving as an advisory-director to the board of directors.

Neurobiological Foundations for EMDR Practice

URI BERGMANN, PhD

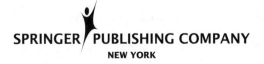

SPRINGER PUBLISHING COMPANY

NEW YORK

Springer Publishing Company, LLC
11 West 42nd Street
New York, NY 10036
www.springerpub.com

Acquisitions Editor: Sheri W. Sussman
Production Editor: Joseph Stubenrauch
Composition: The Manila Typesetting Company

ISBN: 978-0-8261-0937-8
E-book ISBN: 978-0-8261-0938-5

12 13 14 15/ 5 4 3 2 1

The author and the publisher of this Work have made every effort to use sources believed to be reliable to provide information that is accurate and compatible with the standards generally accepted at the time of publication. The author and publisher shall not be liable for any special, consequential, or exemplary damages resulting, in whole or in part, from the readers' use of, or reliance on, the information contained in this book. The publisher has no responsibility for the persistence or accuracy of URLs for external or third-party Internet Web sites referred to in this publication and does not guarantee that any content on such Web sites is, or will remain, accurate or appropriate.

Library of Congress Cataloging-in-Publication Data
Bergmann, Uri.
  Neurobiological foundations for EMDR practice / Uri Bergmann.
     p. ; cm.
  Neurobiological foundations for eye movement desensitization and reprocessing practice
  Includes bibliographical references and index.
  ISBN 978-0-8261-0937-8 (alk. paper) -- ISBN 978-0-8261-0938-5 (e-book)
  I. Title. II. Title: Neurobiological foundations for eye movement desensitization and reprocessing practice.
  [DNLM: 1. Eye Movement Desensitization Reprocessing. 2. Consciousness--physiology. 3. Nervous System Physiological Phenomena. WM 425.5.D4]
  LCclassification not assigned
  612.8--dc23

2012012019

Printed in the United States of America by Bang Printing

To my family,
the source of my purpose, pride, joy, and inspiration.

Contents

Preface

Henry David Thoreau wrote, "Do not worry if you have built your castles in the air. They are where they should be. Now put the foundations under them." This notion of dreaming and then following your imaginings has been the impetus for this book, an undertaking dedicated to constructing a neurobiological foundation for eye movement desensitization and reprocessing (EMDR) practice and research by integrating various research bases that have not, as yet, found themselves equally and comprehensively addressed in a published work. Twenty years of EMDR practice has made it undeniably apparent that in order to truly understand, practice, and research this astonishing and mysterious form of psychotherapy, one needs to be aware of and appreciate the neural mechanisms underlying consciousness and information processing, human development and attachment, disorders of information processing that manifest in the majority of the psychopathology treated by clinicians, trauma and dissociation, and the relationship of stress and trauma on immune function and health.

Given that EMDR is so profoundly guided by an information-processing model, it is crucial to examine how it measures up to researched neurobiological models of consciousness and information processing. The more that this model is seen to be consistent with neurobiological research (illustrated in later chapters), the more the model will be bolstered and grounded.

The best way to generate truly comprehensive neurobiological theoretical models of EMDR, which provide the best blueprints for research, is through a comprehensive consideration and understanding of the neural underpinnings of information processing. If we can ask how EMDR's sensory stimulation and treatment protocol impact the central neural circuitry of information processing and facilitate its repair, we can generate detailed theories that are more amenable to research.

For centuries, society has recoiled from the notion that trauma and neglect are pervasive. A great deal of confusion exists in both our society and our profession regarding trauma, the extent and pervasiveness of familial neglect, and the nature of dissociative processes. Rather than understanding that our history as a human race is profoundly traumatic, we choose to believe that we have survived and adapted. We apply the same lack of vision to our children, believing that come what may, they are resilient.

Within our various professions, academicians at the most prestigious universities tell us that traumatic and dissociative disorders are the creations of suggestive therapists and false memory syndromes. We in the traumatology community try to shed light on this darkness, but psychological and phenomenological explanations are insufficient. It is only through a neurobiological understanding that our ideas will be given the utmost credibility. We must, with respect to our practice, be able to understand and also illustrate clearly to others that the unusual and often bizarre symptoms that we label as traumatic and dissociative disorders are the outcomes of dysregulated, evolutionarily based, neural action systems that are completely predicated by the nature of the attachment between infants and their caretakers. This can be accomplished only by a neurobiological foundation that informs our understanding of human development, attachment, disorders of attachment, and information processing.

Finally, given the myriad manifestations of somatic symptoms and medical illnesses that many of our patients present with, understanding the relationship between stress, trauma, and immune function is imperative. It is crucial that we understand and are able to differentiate somatic or somatoform symptoms from the immunoinflammatory illnesses, which are now referred to as *medically unexplained symptoms*, such as fibromyalgia, systemic lupus erythematosus, reflex sympathetic dystrophy, Hashimoto thyroiditis, Graves' disease, chronic fatigue syndrome, and others, which will be detailed in this book.

Understanding these illnesses and their differentiation from other somatoform symptoms has its greatest import with respect to treatment implications. Somatic symptoms, often conceptualized as manifestations of trauma in the body, are often effectively targeted and treated with EMDR, as part of a comprehensive and phased trauma treatment. However, patients presenting with psychological difficulties (whether or not trauma related) and medically unexplained symptoms must also be referred for treatment to endocrinologists, oncologists, or immunologists in order to attempt to reregulate the hyperimmune function in these patients, which is apparently causative with respect to their illnesses.

It is my hope that the information presented in this writing will be received as informative and clearly integrated, while the presentation of the subject matter provides for an ease of understanding.

Acknowledgments

First and foremost, I would like to begin by saluting and thanking Francine Shapiro for lighting and spreading the flame of eye movement desensitization and reprocessing (EMDR), a fire at which we and our patients have warmed ourselves and, thereby, grown.

I would also like to express my enormous admiration and gratitude to Robbie Dunton, Francine Shapiro's right hand from the beginning, throughout the development of EMDR, and in the founding and continuance of the EMDR Institute.

To Sheri Sussman, executive editor at Springer Publishing, I would like to express my admiration and immense gratitude for her colossal assistance in the organization and editing of this book.

My profound thanks go to Tom Jennings for his invaluable assistance with major portions of the manuscript.

I would also like to thank my wife, Sherrill, and daughter, Danielle, for their vital creative assistance with portions of this book.

Finally, I would like to honor the spirit of my father, Berthold Bergmann, a dedicated physician whose lifelong amazement at the wonders of physiology and neurobiology infuse every aspect of my professional curiosity and every page of this book.

CHAPTER 1

Introduction

The human mind is difficult to investigate, but the biological foundations of the mind, especially consciousness, are generally regarded as the most daunting. Antonio Damasio (1999) has argued that if elucidating the nature of the mind is the last frontier of the life sciences, consciousness often seems like the last mystery in the illumination of the mind. He notes,

> The matter of mind, in general, and of consciousness in particular, allows humans to exercise to the vanishing point, the desire for understanding and the appetite for wonderment at their own nature that Aristotle recognized as so distinctively human. What could be more difficult to know than to know how we know? What could be more dizzying than to realize that it is our having consciousness which makes possible and even inevitable our questions about consciousness? (p. 4)

Echoing this sentiment, Alan Hobson (2009) opines that "consciousness, we are relieved to admit, is finally a bona fide subject of inquiry. Let us take the first obvious step and teach it to study itself" (p. xi).

For Rodolfo Llinas (2001), consciousness is a function of mindness, driving him to ask,

> Why is mindness so mysterious to us? Why has it always been this way? The processes that generate such states as thinking, consciousness, and dreaming are foreign to us, I fancy, because they always seem to be generated with no apparent relation to the external world. They seem impalpably internal. (p. 4)

Similarly, Alan Hobson (2009) observes,

> The brain still tends to keep most of its activity out of consciousness, but what it excludes or admits is governed more by rules of activation, neuromodulation, input–output gating than by the predominance of repression. The unconscious is now seen as a useful lookup system for the conscious brain rather than a seething source of devils aiming at the disruption of consciousness. Consciousness itself is, thus, a tool for the investigation of itself as well as for the study of that part of the unconscious that is dynamically repressed. (p. xi)

Throughout his writings, Sigmund Freud articulated his ideas through the organizing concepts of the "self" and the "object." For Freud, the people interacting with the *self* were the *objects* of the self's drives and desires. Ironically, neuroscientists today tend to view consciousness, from its basic levels to its utmost complexity, as the integrated neural function that brings together the object and the self.

Accordingly, Damasio (1999) opines,

> At its elemental and most basic level, consciousness lets us recognize an irresistible urge to stay alive and experience a concern for the self. At its most profound and elaborate level, consciousness helps us develop a concern for other selves and improve the art of life. (p. 5)

Evolution, over these millions of years has given rise to our complex brain and, somehow, through the interactions among its 100 billion neurons, connected by trillions of synapses, our conscious experience of the world and of ourselves emerges.

Like it or not, consciousness is the pivotal biological function that allows us to know sorrow and joy, suffering and pleasure, embarrassment and pride, and grief and reunion. Damasio (1999) muses, "Do not blame Eve for knowing; blame consciousness, and thank it, too" (p. 4).

CONSCIOUSNESS AND EMDR

Consciousness and EMDR have been intimately related, albeit under a different name. Whereas the field of neurobiology has utilized the term *consciousness* to denote the processes of sensation, perception, learning, cognition, emotion, somatosensory integration, and memory; the discipline of psychology has chosen to use the term *information processing*. Accordingly, they will be used interchangeably. If we tend to favor the term *consciousness* in this book, it is only because it feels more human.

Throughout the past 20 years, EMDR has evolved into a therapeutic approach guided by the adaptive information processing (AIP) model (Shapiro, 2001). In 1990, the name change from *eye movement desensitization* to *eye movement desensitization and reprocessing* heralded a change in orientation from the initial behavioral formulation of simple desensitization of anxiety to a more integrated information processing paradigm. This evolution ushered in the accelerated information processing model, which illustrated a clinically grounded understanding of the underlying principles that govern perception and the integration of new information within cognitive, memorial, and emotional frameworks (Shapiro, 1995). In 2001, this continued evolution brought us the aforementioned adaptive information processing model. Regarding these models, Francine Shapiro (2001) has argued that "their utility lies in their ability not only to explain, but to predict clinical outcomes" (p. 14).

As we shall see, as this book develops, consciousness and EMDR are inextricably intertwined, giving us an information processing paradigm that provides an integrated approach that can incorporate and interpret key aspects of such diverse modalities as psychodynamic, behavioral, cognitive, gestalt, ego-state, and body-oriented therapies. If the neurobiology of consciousness enables our understanding of the neural interrelationship between self and object, EMDR has given us both tools and mysteries to solve in the repair of the self and its relation to its objects.

THE PROGRESS OF SCIENCE

Reflecting on the foregoing, it becomes apparent that the understanding of the human mind in biological terms has emerged as one of the most important challenges for science in the 21st century. Our goal in this endeavor has been to understand the biological underpinnings of sensation, perception, cognition, learning, memory, emotion, and sensory integration.

The progress that researchers have made in the field of neuroscience, unthinkable even a few decades ago, has made possible our present understanding. The discovery of the structure of DNA in 1953 revolutionized biology, giving it a foundational framework for comprehending the mechanisms underlying the gene's ability to control the functioning of cells. This breakthrough led to a basic understanding of gene regulation and gene-related cell function, propelling an understanding of the science of biology to a level rivaling that of physics and chemistry.

Imbued with this knowledge, biology turned its focus to its loftiest goal, the understanding of the biological nature of the human mind. This endeavor, once considered to be prescientific and impossible, has achieved great momentum and growth. Ironically, these new insights did not come from the disciplines traditionally concerned with mind, from philosophy or psychology. Instead, they evolved from the merger of these disciplines with the biology of the brain, a new synthesis made possible by the remarkable achievements in molecular biology. The result has been a new science of mind, a science that has harnessed the power of molecular biology to examine the great remaining mysteries of life.

MIND AND BRAIN

This new science is grounded by five principles. First, mind and brain are inseparable. The brain is a multifaceted biological organ of vast computational abilities that constructs our sensory experiences, regulates our thoughts and emotions, and mediates our actions. Our brain is responsible not only for motor behaviors such as running and eating but also for the complex and multifaceted acts considered quintessentially human, such as thinking, speaking, and creating works of art.

Second, each mental function in the brain, from the simplest reflexes to the most creative acts in language, music, and art, is carried out by specialized neural circuits throughout different regions of the brain. It has been noted by many in the neuroscience community that it is preferable to use the term *biology of mind* to refer to the set of mental operations carried out by these specialized neural circuits rather than *biology of the mind*, which can be seen to inaccurately connote that there is a unique or singular place, a single location in the brain, that carries out mental operations.

Third, all of these circuits are composed of the same elementary signaling units, the neuron. Fourth, these neural circuits use specific molecules to generate signals within and between nerve cells. Finally, the specific signaling molecules have been conserved and retained through millions of years of evolution. Some of them were present in the cells of our most ancient ancestors and can be found today in our most distant and primitive evolutionary relatives.

Hence, we gain from this new knowledge regarding the science of mind not only insights into ourselves—how we perceive, learn, remember, feel, and act—but also a new viewpoint of ourselves within the context of biological evolution. Accordingly, this allows us to appreciate that the human mind evolved from molecules used by our most primitive ancestors and that the extraordinary conservation of the molecular mechanisms that regulate life's various processes also applies to our mental life.

In a similar vein, the search for EMDR's mechanisms of action began in the early 1990s, initially proceeding slowly and tentatively. As we entered the new millennium, the pace quickened. Theoretically driven speculative models, grounded in empirical findings from related neurobiological research bases, became more detailed and prevalent. In parallel, neurobiological studies became increasingly widespread, utilizing psychophysiological and neuroimaging examinations of EMDR treatment.

In the past decade, it has become increasingly apparent that people lacking a background in science are as enthusiastic to learn about this new knowledge regarding the science of mind and consciousness as scientists are to explain it.

SCIENTIFIC GROWTH OF EMDR

A similar phenomenon can be seen in the EMDR world. In the beginning, few were interested in the neurobiology of EMDR. A talk speculating on EMDR's neural mechanisms would attract 30 people, on a good day. As in other aspects of neuroscience, this interest has exploded. Hundreds are now in attendance at EMDR workshops currently held worldwide, solely focused on the topic of the neurobiology of EMDR. Hence, these occurrences have made it apparent that nonscientists are prepared to make the effort to understand the key issues of brain science if scientists are willing to make the effort to explain them.

OUTLINE OF THE BOOK

Thus, this book is written both technically and as an introduction to the neural underpinnings of consciousness and EMDR. These knowledge bases have emerged from theories and observations and have evolved into the experimental science of today. Pertinent neuroscience research relative to our understanding of consciousness, information processing, and traumatic disorders of consciousness will be reviewed and examined.

The reader will first be presented with basic research in the neurosciences relevant to online/wakeful information processing, which includes sensation, perception, somatosensory integration, cognition, memory, emotion, language, and motricity (motor function). In addition, offline/sleep information processing will be examined with respect to slow-wave sleep and cognitive memorial processing as well as REM/dream sleep and its function in emotional and semantic memory processing.

The second section will examine the neuroscience research relevant to disorders of consciousness, which includes (in brief) anesthesia, coma, and other neurological disorders. Major focus will be given to the disorders of type I posttraumatic stress disorder (PTSD), complex PTSD/dissociative disorders, and personality disorders.

The reader, in the third section, will be presented with an examination of neuroscience research relevant to chronic trauma and autoimmune function. Particularly, a number of medical illnesses, collectively known as medically unexplained symptoms, will be examined, which include fibromyalgia, chronic fatigue syndrome, reflex sympathetic dystrophy, systemic lupus erythematosus, and rheumatoid arthritis. These disorders will be examined from the perspective of autoimmune hyperactivity resulting from the unusual neuroendocrine profile of persons with PTSD.

The fourth and final section will examine the foregoing material with respect to the adaptive information processing model. Treatment implications vis-à-vis the various types of PTSD and the presentations of medically unexplained symptoms will be explored in detail.

To the reader who is fluent in this material, it will become immediately apparent that my thinking has been greatly influenced by the works of Antonio Damasio, Rodolfo Llinas, Jaak Panksepp, and Allan Schore. Their empirical and descriptive writings have enabled me to extract form out of the empirical chaos that has engulfed the study of consciousness and information processing.

CHAPTER 2

What Is Consciousness?

THE MYSTERY OF CONSCIOUSNESS

How, then, does the brain's internal activity actually represent the external world? How does it allow us to interact with the external world and internally with our own? How can it manage to differentiate external from internal reality? If consciousness is intrinsic to brain function, then is there some sort of place within the brain that we can isolate as being the seat of consciousness, or do we have to look more for a neural network distributed over a larger scale, throughout the brain?

An alternative way of exploring these mysteries is to ask how the brain mediates information processing, taking us to the study of individual neurons and their relationship to neural systems. Individual neurons function together in specialized groups, or systems, each serving a specific function. Systems neuroscience is the study of these neural systems, which include those involved in vision, memory, language, emotion, and motor function. Accordingly, these systems possess common properties, particularly in that they all process high-order information regarding our environment and biological needs. Consequently, the study of systems neuroscience places paramount emphasis on the identification of the neural structures and events associated with the hierarchical steps in information processing. Hence, we can now refine our questions further and ask the following: How is information encoded (sensation)? How is it interpreted to confer meaning (perception)? How is it modified or stored (learning and memory)? How is it used to predict the future state of the environment and the consequences of action (decision making/emotion)? How is it used to guide behavior (motor control) and to communicate (language)?

The 20th century has witnessed incredible progress in understanding these processes. This ascending growth of modern systems neuroscience is resultant, in part, to the convergence of three key subdisciplines, each of which contributed major technical or conceptual advances to the understanding of information processing.

Neuropsychology: Localization of the Biological Source of Mental Function

An initial question one might ask about an information processing device regards its gross structure and the relationship between structural elements and their functions. The earliest approach to this question and the approach that has best withstood the test of time has been to observe the behavioral or psychological consequences of localized lesions of brain tissue. The modern discipline of neuropsychology was founded on this approach, drawing both from clinical case studies of brain injuries sustained in battle and from experimental studies of the effects of targeted destruction of brain tissue in animals. Consequently, the functions of specific brain regions, such as those involved in sensation, perception, memory, and language, have been inferred.

Neuroanatomy: Patterns of Connectivity in Information Processing Stages

The Neuron Doctrine

Modern neural science, as we now know it, began when Santiago Ramon y Cajal (1899) provided the critical evidence for the "neuron doctrine," the idea that neurons served as the functional signaling units of the nervous system and that neurons connect to one another in precise ways (Albright, Jessel, Kandel, & Posner, 2001). Ramon y Cajal's neuron doctrine (which is considered more broadly at a later point) represented a major shift in emphasis to a cellular view of the brain. Utilizing the histological cellular staining techniques developed by him and Camillo Golgi (which earned both the Nobel Prize in Physiology or Medicine in 1906), Ramon y Cajal observed that neurons were discrete cells, bounded by their membranes, and inferred that nerve cells communicate with one another only at specialized points of opposition, contact points that Charles Sherrington (1906) was later to name *synapses*. Ramon y Cajal evidenced an uncanny ability to infer from static cellular images remarkable functional insights into the dynamic properties of neurons.

Dynamic Polarization

One of Ramon y Cajal's most remarkable insights was the principle of dynamic polarization. According to this principle, electrical signaling within neurons is unidirectional. Consequently, signals propagate from the receiving pole of the neuron, through the dendrites and the cell body to the axon, and then along the axon to the output pole of the neuron, the presynaptic axon terminal. The principle of dynamic polarization proved enormously influential in that it provided the first functionally coherent view of the various compartments of neurons. In addition, by identifying the directionality of information flow in the nervous system, dynamic polarization provided a logic and set of rules for mapping the individual components of pathways in the brain that constitute a coherent neural circuit. Thus, in contrast to Golgi's chaotic view of the nervous system, which conceived of the brain as a diffuse nerve net in which every imaginable type of interaction appeared possible, Ramon y Cajal's brilliant experimental analysis and observations heralded today's modern understanding of neural function and the brain's most important function, the processing of information (Albright et al., 2001).

Neural Structure

The discipline of neuroanatomy, which blossomed at the turn of the century following the adoption of the neuron doctrine and which has benefited from many subsequent technical advances, has revealed much about the fine structure of the brain's components and the manner in which they are connected to one another. As was noted, one of the earliest and most influential technical developments was the discovery by Golgi and Ramon y Cajal of methods for selective staining of individual neurons, which permitted their visualization by light microscopy. As a result, it became possible to identify differences in the morphology (form and structure) of cells in different brain regions as markers for functional diversity. This procedure, known as cytoarchitectonics, was promoted energetically in the early decades of the 20th century by the anatomists Korbinian Brodmann and Oscar and Cecile Vogt. Brodmann's cytoarchitectonic map of the human cerebral cortex, which was published in 1909 and charted the positions of some 50 distinct cortical zones, has served as a guidebook for generations of scientists and clinicians and as a catalyst for countless studies of cortical functional organization (Albright et al., 2001).

Neural Connectivity

Arguably the most significant outcome of the ability to label neurons was the capability to trace connections between diverse brain regions. Consequently, cell-labeling techniques have undergone vast refinement over the past three decades. Small amounts of fluorescent or radioactive substances, for instance, can now be injected with precision into one brain region and subsequently detected in other regions, providing evidence for connectivity. The products of anatomical tract tracing are wiring diagrams (neural maps) of major brain systems, which are continuously evolving in their accuracy and completeness and have been crucial to the investigation of information flow throughout the brain and for understanding the hierarchy of information processing stages.

Neurophysiology: Uncovering Cellular Representations of the World

Acceptance of the neuron doctrine and recognition of the electrical nature of nervous tissue ushered in an understanding of the information represented by neurons as a result of their intrinsic (basic internal) electrical properties.

Electrical Recordings

Methods of amplification and recording of small electrical potentials were developed in the 1920s by Edgar Adrian. This innovative technology of electroencephalography allowed neurobiologists to relate a neuronal signal directly to a specific event, such as the representation of a sensory stimulus, and became a cornerstone of systems neuroscience. By the 1930s, electrophysiological methods were adequately refined to permit recordings to be made from individual neurons. Sensory processing and motor control evolved as natural targets for study. Albright et al. (2001) note that the great successes of single-neuron electrophysiology are most evident from the work of Vernon Mountcastle in the somatosensory system and David Hubel and Torsten Wiesel in the visual cortex, whose investigations, commencing in the late 1950s, greatly shaped our understanding of the relationship between neuronal and sensory events.

Neuroimaging

In the 1970s, cognitive psychology, the science of mind, merged with neuroscience, the science of the brain. The result was cognitive neuroscience, the discipline that introduced biological methods of exploring mental processes to modern cognitive psychology. In the 1980s, cognitive neuroscience was enhanced and energized by the advent of functional neuroimaging. This technology enabled brain scientists to peer inside the human brain, observing the activity of various neural regions as subjects engaged in higher mental functions, such as perception, thought, memory, and motor function. The 1980s also ushered in the use of magnetoencephalography (MEG), facilitating the examination of neural network and system activation, throughout the entire brain, simultaneously, in real time.

Collectively, these three areas of neuroscience comprise a revolutionary experimental arsenal, which has already uncovered, empirically or in outline structure, operational mechanisms and functions of vast neural systems, such as those implicated in the mediation of vision, memory, motricity (motor function), cognition, emotion, somatosensory integration, and language.

Consciousness and Evolution

Eric Kandel (2006) has argued that every revolution has its origins in the past and that the revolution that culminated in the new science of mind is no exception. Although the central role of biology in the study of mental or psychological processes was new, the profound ability of biology to influence the way we see ourselves was not. In the mid-19th century, Charles Darwin argued that we were not uniquely created but rather evolved gradually from lower animal ancestors. He proposed the even more daring idea that evolution's driving force was not a conscious, intelligent, or divine purpose but a "blind" process of natural selection, a completely mechanistic sorting process of random trial and error (a tinkering) based on hereditary variations.

Darwin's ideas challenged the teaching of most religions. Because biology's original purpose had been to explain the divine design of nature, his ideas shredded the historic bond between religion and biology. Eric Kandel (2006) notes that consequently, for some, the neurobiology of mind is potentially more disturbing because it suggests that not only the body but also mind and the specific molecules that underlie our highest mental processes, of consciousness of self and others and of the past and future, have evolved from our animal ancestors. Nonetheless, as we shall see later in this book, this evolutionary perspective has profoundly facilitated our understanding by guiding us to study the nervous systems of lower animals, such as the mollusk Aplysia. By studying learning, such as habituation, sensitization, and conditioning in this animal, the neural patterns of learning and memory were clearly and consistently codified for the first time. With time and increased sophistications in technology, similar neural patterns were discovered in human functioning, confirming both Darwin's ideas of evolutionary connectedness and Ramon y Cajal's theories of synaptic plasticity.

Characteristics of Consciousness

In the past 20 years, consciousness has also been described and investigated with respect to three characteristics: unity, subjectivity, and prediction.

Unity of Consciousness

The unitary nature of consciousness refers to the fact that our experiences come to us as a unified whole. All of the various sensory modalities (i.e., color, shape, depth, sound, taste, and smell) are integrated and melded into a single, coherent conscious experience.

Subjectivity

The foregoing speaks to information that comes to us from the outside world. The same, however, is also true of our inner proprioceptive experiences, wherein modalities such as associations, memories, and emotions are likewise integrated and melded with our sensory experiences to produce a coherent subjective experience. We consider this issue more broadly and in more detail later in the book.

Prediction

Regarding prediction, it has been noted by Llinas (2001) that consciousness, or the mindness state, which may or may not represent external reality (subjective states, imagining or dreaming), has

> evolved as the goal-oriented device that implements predicted/intentional interactions between a living organism and its environment. Such transactions, to be successful, require an inherited, prewired instrument that generates an internal subjective image of the external world that can be compared with sensory transduced objective information from the external environment. (p. 3)

Given that this functional comparison of internally generated sensorimotor images, with real-time sensory information from the organism's immediate environment, is defined as perception, then the function of the underlying workings of perception is to mediate *prediction*, that is, "the useful expectation of events yet to come" (p. 3). From an evolutionary/survival perspective, which is the driving force that all species have in common, prediction, with its goal-oriented essence, is at the very core of brain function and consciousness. Obviously, the ability to predict is critical in the animal kingdom; a creature's life depends upon it. Still, the mechanism of prediction is far more ubiquitous in the brain's control of body functions.

Prediction at Work

Consider the simple act of reaching for a carton of milk in the refrigerator. Without giving much thought to our actions, we must predict the carton's weight, its slipperiness, its degree of fullness, and finally, the compensatory balance we must apply for a successful smooth trajectory of the contents of the carton into our glass.

The brain's predictive ability can also be generated in the absence of conscious awareness. As an example, have you ever found yourself blinking just before a bug lands in your eye? You did not observe the bug, at least on a conscious level, yet you, somehow, predicted the event and blinked appropriately to prevent its entry into your eye. Prediction is at the heart of this protective mechanism (Llinas, 2001).

Prediction, continually operative at conscious, unconscious, and reflexive levels, is pervasive throughout most if not all levels of brain function. As we shall see later, in order for the nervous system to predict, it must perform a rapid comparison of the sensory properties/input of the external world with a separate internal/subjective representation of the world. In humans (and a number of animals), this internal representation is driven by sensorimotor experiences, associations, memories, and emotions. This precarious balance of outer objectivity and inner subjectivity and the predictions that it generates about ourselves, our environment, and those around us is at the heart of our knowledge, creativity, joys and sorrows, and the quality of our relationships.

Prediction and EMDR

As we shall see later in this book, prediction and information processing also hold a crucial place in EMDR treatment, given the centrality of the negative and positive cognitions, both of which articulate predictions regarding the environment, others/objects, and the self. Accordingly, a distorted negative cognition is clearly symptomatic of maladaptive predictive information processing.

In all these permutations of consciousness and information processing, oscillating neural systems, which correspond to the various outer sensory and inner proprioceptive modalities, are synchronized with respect to their oscillations to produce coherent (unified) conscious experiences. We shall return in broad detail to this issue, known as temporal binding, throughout the book as we examine consciousness, disorders of consciousness, and EMDR.

CHAPTER 3

Cellular Communication

THE NEURAL ENVIRONMENT

Our brain has the consistency of firm jelly and is, consequently, protectively encased in a thick bony skull. The brain literally floats in about 150 ml of cerebrospinal fluid (CSF) secreted by the choroid plexus. Approximately 500 ml of CSF is secreted daily, which slowly circulates throughout the brain and exits into the cerebral veins through the arachnoid villi. The brain has no lymphatic lubricating system, so the CSF serves as a partial substitute (Kandel, 1991a). Such is the environment of the neural cell.

Origin of Neurons

Neurons, the nerve cells that make up the brain, are signaling devices of a rather remarkable kind, constituting a significant evolutionary specialization of the eukaryotic (elementary basic animal) cell, which allowed for the evolution of natural "computation" by cellular ensembles (Kandel, 1991a; Llinas, 2001). In other words, in order for evolution to create the brain, the transformation from basic eukaryotic cells into neuronal cells was required. Consequently, the signaling capabilities of neurons underlie all aspects of our mental life, from sensory perception to control of movement, including the generation of thought, memory, and the experience and expression of emotion. Understanding the signaling properties of neurons, therefore, is essential for understanding the biological basis of any aspect of information processing.

As was noted above, our initial insights into how signaling occurs in the brain date back to the end of the 19th century and especially to the extraordinary contributions of Santiago Ramon y Cajal (1899). It was Ramon y Cajal who first observed that the nerve cells in all animals have surprisingly similar anatomical features. As a result of this finding, we now know that the different learning capabilities of different animals are related not so much to the type of nerve cells that an animal has in its brain but rather to the number of nerve cells and the way that they are interconnected.

With few exceptions, the larger the number of nerve cells, and the more intricate their pattern of interconnection, the greater will be an animal's capability for diverse and complex types of learning. For example, snails have approximately 20,000 neurons in their brains. Fruit flies have approximately 300,000 nerve cells. Mice can have as many as 10 billion neurons and humans an excess of 100 billion neural cells. In humans, each neuron in the brain, in turn, can make approximately 1,000 connections, at any given time, to other neurons at specialized connecting junctions called synapses (Squire & Kandel, 1999).

While we reflect on the vast number of neurons, it is worth noting that glia cells outnumber neurons in our central nervous system by a ratio of 50:1. Glia (or glial cells) are the cells that provide support to the neurons. In much the same way that the foundation, framework, walls, and roof of a house provide the structure through which run the various electrical, cable, and telephone lines, along with various pipes for water and waste, not only do glial cells provide the structural framework that allows networks of neurons to remain connected, they also attend to the brain's various housekeeping functions (such as neuronal nutrition, the formation of myelin, and removal of debris after neuronal death).

Neuronal Structure

Structurally, every neuron has four components: a cell body, a number of dendrites, an axon, and a group of axon terminations called presynaptic terminals (see Figure 3.1).

The cell body is the large spherical central portion of the neuron, containing the nucleus, which, in turn, houses the DNA that encodes the neuron's genes. Surrounding the nucleus is the cytoplasm, a liquid sap-like substance that contains a variety of molecular machinery (structures) necessary for the cell to function. The cell body gives rise to two types of long slender threads, or extensions, generically known as nerve cells processes and specifically known as the dendrites and the axon. The dendrites typically consist of elaborately branching processes (extensions) that extend from the cell body, often in the form of tree branches, and form the input components or receptive area for incoming signals from other neurons. The axon, the output component of the neuron, is a tubular process that extends from the cell body. Depending on the neuron's specific function, the axon can travel distances as short as 0.1 mm to as long as a meter or more. Near its ending, the axon divides into many fine branches, each of which has a specialized terminal region called the presynaptic terminal. The presynaptic terminals contact the specialized receptive surfaces (dendrites) of other cells. Through this contact at the synapse, the nerve cell transmits information about its activity to other neurons or to organs such as muscles or glands (Kandel, 1991; Squire & Kandel, 1999).

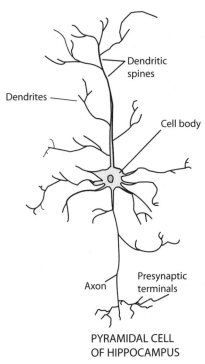

Dendritic
spines

Dendrites

Cell body

Presynaptic
Axon   terminals

PYRAMIDAL CELL
OF HIPPOCAMPUS

FIGURE 3.1   Regardless of their shape, all neurons contain dendrites, a cell body, axons, and presynaptic terminals.

Based on Ramon y Cajal's formulation of dynamic polarization, we now know that neural information flows in a predictable and consistent direction within each nerve cell. Information is received at the dendrites and into the cell body, and then from these receiving sites, information is conveyed to the axon, from the axon to the presynaptic terminals, and onward to the next neuron.

Neuronal Voltage

A neuron is in many ways like a battery, and like a battery, it generates voltage. This voltage is known as the membrane potential. Neurons, like all living cells, are surrounded by a plasma membrane that is impermeable to outside ions (negatively and positively charged atoms). Consequently, this property allows a neuron to maintain different concentrations of ions between the inside and the outside of the cell. In a typical mammalian neuron, there is a large difference in the concentration of ions [positively charged (sodium and potassium) and negatively charged (chlorine) atoms] between the intracellular (inside) and extracellular (outside) environments. In addition, the interior of the neuron has a high concentration of large negatively charged proteins. We will return to this in increasing detail throughout this chapter.

Plasma Membrane

The plasma membrane (the neuron's outer casing), composed of lipids (a broad group of naturally occurring molecules, which includes fats, waxes, and fat-soluble vitamins), prevents the diffusion of ions across the membrane. Therefore, the only way that ions can cross this barrier (either out of or into the neuron) is through specialized *channels* or *gates*. These channels are essentially transmembrane pores that permit the movement of particular ions while excluding others. Accordingly, such channels can be in either an open or a closed state. When a neuron is at rest, most ion channels are closed. However, potassium and sodium channels can sometimes be ever-so-slightly open, allowing for a minuscule leakage of potassium ions out of the cell and sodium ions into the cell, ostensibly, to fine-tune voltage.

In a typical neuron, the internal concentration of positively charged potassium is higher than the external concentration, whereas the internal concentration of positively charged sodium ions is markedly lower than the external concentration. In addition, as noted above, the interior of the neuron has a high concentration of large negatively charged proteins. Therefore, the separation of ions, inside relative to the outside of the neuron, mediates and maintains differences in voltage (Kandel, Siegelbaum, & Schwartz, 1991). We return to this, repeatedly, in layered detail.

Electrical and Chemical Gradients

Opposites attract. Therefore, positively charged ions seek a negative environment, whereas negatively charged ions seek a positive environment, in each case moving toward electrical neutrality. This is the *electrical* part of the ionic movement gradient (force of movement).

Ions also have a preference for equal concentrations. Therefore, if the concentration of sodium ions, for example, is higher on one side of the membrane, sodium ions will, if given access, cross the membrane in an attempt to equalize the distribution. This is the *chemical* part of the ionic movement gradient (Koester, 1991; Llinas, 2001). Consequently, the combined electrical drive and concentration differences inside with respect to the outside of the cell determine ionic directional flow. Whether or not the ions will flow is predicated by issues of permeability, that is, whether the ionic channels are open or closed.

Ionic Channels/Gates

If the cell membrane's ionic channel is open, it represents a path for specific ions to move across. This channel, therefore, is considered to be specifically permeable to a particular type of ion. Therefore, if the channel is closed, it becomes impermeable to that particular ion. Consequently, the size of the membrane current is determined by the rate of movement of ions through their respective channels. This rate is mediated by three occurrences: first, the respective channels must be open; second, the appropriate ion species for the open channel must be present; and third, there must exist a driving force acting on the given ion (it will move down its electrochemical gradients).

Neural Signaling

Neurons utilize two types of signals: They employ an "all-or-none" action potential for signaling within the neuron for passing information from one region or compartment of the neuron to the other (such as from the dendrites to the cell body and from the cell body to the axon and the presynaptic terminals). Additionally, they utilize a "graded" synaptic potential to pass information from one cell to another through the process of synaptic transmission. We revisit this in detail below.

Resting Potential

Before exploring the action and synaptic potentials, we need to consider the resting potential, which is the baseline condition upon which all other cellular signals are expressed. The external plasma membrane of the neuron maintains, at rest, an internal electrical difference of about 70 mini-volts (mV), relative to the voltage outside the cell. This is the resting potential. It results from the unequal distribution of sodium, potassium, and other ions across the nerve cell membrane, such that the inside of the cell membrane is markedly negatively charged in relation to the outside. Given that the outside of the membrane is arbitrarily defined as 0 mV, we can, therefore, state that the resting membrane potential is approximately –70 mV. In describing this situation, we could say that there is a polar difference between the inner and outer voltages. Accordingly, when at resting potential, the neuron is considered to be *polarized*.

Changes in Polarization

Action potentials and synaptic potentials result from perturbations (disturbances) of the cell membrane, induced by incoming synaptic potentials from nearby neurons that cause the membrane potential to increase or decrease. Therefore, an increase in membrane potential, say from –70 to –80 mV, is referred to as *hyperpolarization*, whereas a reduction in membrane potential, from –70 to +10 mV, is referred to as *depolarization*. As we shall see in detail below, depolarization increases the cell's ability to generate an action potential and is considered to be excitatory. Conversely, hyperpolarization makes it less likely that a cell will generate an action potential and is, therefore, considered as inhibitory.

Action Potential

The action potential is an electrical signal resulting from the depolarization of the neuron that travels from the dendrites and cell body of the neuron, along the entire length of the axon, to its presynaptic terminals, where the neuron contacts another nerve cell. Action potentials derive their name from the fact that they are signals that propagate actively along the axon (Squire & Kandel, 1999).

Depolarization

When a neuron is stimulated by the neurotransmission of another neuron, it results in a brief opening of the sodium channels and a slight inward infusion of positively charged sodium ions, causing its membrane potential to become slightly more positive (from –70 to –50 mV). This is referred to as a *partial depolarization* and is preparatory for the *full depolarization*. This is followed by a complete depolarization, wherein sodium channels open fully, thereby allowing positively charged sodium ions to rapidly diffuse into the cell. As a result, the inside of the membrane voltage briefly becomes more positive than the outside (+20 mV), is considered depolarized, and facilitates the firing of the action potential.

Repolarization

This is followed by the closing of the sodium channels. The potassium channels now open. Repelled by the positive charge inside the neuron (the electrical gradient), positively charged potassium ions now diffuse through the potassium channels to the outside. This outward movement of potassium ions reduces the positive valence of the inner charge, facilitating the return to the resting negative charge, thereby *repolarizing* the neuron. The potassium channels now close. Before the membrane potential stabilizes again, at about –70 mV, there is a small undershooting in the membrane potential (to approximately –80 mV). During this brief refractory period, the neuron cannot fire another action potential. This is known as the *refractory/recovery potential*. When the membrane potential quickly returns to its resting state/ resting potential (–70 mV), it is now ready to fire another action potential, when necessary (Koester, 1991).

Synapses and Synaptic Transmission

As was noted above, it was Ramon y Cajal (1899) who first appreciated that neurons communicate with one another at highly specialized contact points called synapses. As we shall see, most of the remarkable information-processing activities of the brain emerge from the signaling properties of synapses. This is mediated by the actions of chemical as well as electrical (or electrotonic) synapses and by the interactions of action and synaptic potentials.

Types of Synapses

With respect to this discussion, electrical synapses are utilized to synchronize large numbers of similar neurons (i.e., hippocampal, amygdaloid, auditory, or visual/color), creating synchronized systems. Essentially, this would allow vast numbers of similar neurons to "become as one neuron." Chemical synapses, on the other hand, are generally used for intersystem communications (i.e., hippocampal systems communicating with amygdaloid systems) as well as other nonsynchronous communicative functions (Squire & Kandel, 1999). We will return to this.

Types of Potentials

With respect to the difference between action potentials and synaptic potentials, whereas the signal in the axon (action potential) is large, invariant, and all or none, the signal at the synapse (synaptic potential) is graded and modifiable (Squire & Kandel, 1999). We examine both differences in detail below.

Synaptic Structure

A typical synapse has three components: a presynaptic terminal; a postsynaptic target cell; and a small fluid-filled space between these two processes, separating the two neurons. This space, called the synaptic cleft, is approximately 20 nm (2×10^{-8} m) wide (Squire & Kandel, 1999). The presynaptic terminal of one cell communicates across the synaptic cleft with either the cell body or the dendrites of the postsynaptic target cell.

Chemical Synapses and Cellular Communication

Although biologists understood several of these distinctive features of synaptic transmission by the 1930s, much of our knowledge about neurotransmission and neural communication comes from the work of Bernard Katz (1959a, 1959b, 1971) and his colleagues, who worked out many of the fine details and sequences. As a result, the interrelationship between action potentials, transmitters, and synaptic potentials was, for the first time, clearly and empirically articulated (see Figure 3.2).

From the work of Katz and his colleagues, we now know clearly that the current produced by the action potential in the presynaptic cell cannot jump directly across the synaptic cleft to activate the postsynaptic target cell. Instead, the signal undergoes a major transformation at the synapse. As the

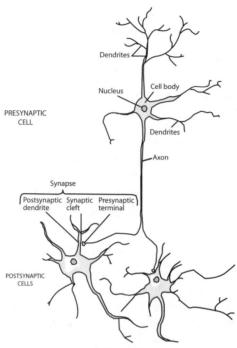

FIGURE 3.2   The long axon branches at its end into numerous presynaptic terminals that form synapses with the dendrites of one or more postsynaptic cells. The presynaptic terminals of a single axon may synapse with as many as 1000 other neurons.

action potential reaches the presynaptic terminals (at the end of the axon), it causes the opening of ion channels for positively charged calcium ions. This causes a large and rapid inward diffusion of calcium ions into the presynaptic terminals. This marked infusion of calcium ions leads to the release of a chemical neurotransmitter.

Katz made his discoveries in the early 1950s, just at the time that researchers began to use the electron microscope to observe nerve cells, allowing for the dissemination of high-resolution pictures of subcellular neural structures. These pictures, in addition to clearly revealing the structures common to all cells, also revealed structures unique to nerve cells.

Neurotransmission

One of Katz's major discoveries was the finding that neurotransmitters are released not as single molecules but as one or more packets of fixed size, each containing approximately 5,000 molecules of the neurotransmitter. Each of these packets is contained in vesicles, which he named *synaptic vesicles*, and is released in an all-or-none fashion. Katz called these packets *quanta* and understood that they were the elementary units of neurotransmitter release.

Relationship of Neurotransmitters and Receptors

Therefore, neurotransmitters diffuse across the synaptic cleft toward the post-synaptic cell, binding to the receptor molecules on the surface of the post-synaptic cell (ion channel area), causing the ion channels (specialized pores on the membrane surface) to widen and open. Ostensibly, the relationship between neurotransmitters and channel receptor sites is that of a key to a lock, respectively. The opening of the ion channels causes the diffusion of positively charged ions (generally sodium) into the postsynaptic cell, which leads to a depolarizing excitatory synaptic potential in the postsynaptic cell, which, if large enough, generates an action potential in that cell (Kandel, 1991b).

Transmitter Reuptake

Chemical neurotransmission ends with the removal of the neurotransmitter from the synaptic cleft. For most neurotransmitters, this occurs through the use of transporters in the presynaptic membrane. Ostensibly, these transporters allow the neurotransmitter molecules to reenter the cell, a process called *reuptake*, which allows them to be recycled for reuse. In other cases, neurotransmitters diffuse away from the synaptic cleft and are eventually degraded by substances such as monoamine oxidase. These same processes are then repeated from neuron to neuron (Kandel, 1991b).

Transmitter Classification

The most common neurotransmitters, relative to this discussion, can be classified into two broad classes. The first group consists of the *amino acids* aspartate, glutamate, gamma-aminobutyric acid, and glycine. The second group consists of the *biogenic amines* acetylcholine, histamine, and serotonin, and the *catecholamines* dopamine, norepinephrine, and epinephrine. There are numerous others, only partially understood and beyond the scope of this discussion.

Excitatory Versus Inhibitory Neurotransmitter Function

Some neurotransmitters are commonly described as "excitatory" or "inhibitory." The only direct effect of a neurotransmitter is to activate one or more types of receptors. The effect on the postsynaptic cell depends, therefore, entirely on the properties of those receptors, that is, do the keys (the neurotransmitters) match the locks (the receptors)?

Excitatory Transmission

It happens that for some neurotransmitters (for example, glutamate), the most important receptors all have excitatory effects, that is, they increase the probability that the target cell will fire an action potential by mediating the depolarization of the target cell. Excitatory neurotransmitters are, therefore, the nervous system's "on switches"; they increase the likelihood that an excitatory signal is sent. Excitatory transmitters can be likened to the accelerator of a car, regulating many of the body's most basic functions, including thought processes, higher thinking, and sympathetic (neuroexcitatory) activity. Physiologically, the excitatory transmitters act as the body's natural stimulants, generally serving to promote wakefulness, energy, and activity.

Inhibitory Transmission

For other neurotransmitters (such as gamma-aminobutyric acid), the most important receptors all have inhibitory effects. Inhibitory neurotransmitters are the nervous system's "*off* switches"; they decrease the likelihood that an excitatory signal will be sent by mediating the hyperpolarization of the target cell. Inhibitory transmitters regulate the activity of the excitatory neurotransmitters, much like the brakes on a car. Physiologically, the inhibitory transmitters act as the body's natural tranquilizers, generally serving to induce sleep, promote calmness, and decrease aggression.

Combined Excitatory and Inhibitory Transmission

There are, however, other neurotransmitters, such as acetylcholine, for which both excitatory and inhibitory receptors exist. In addition, there are some types of receptors that activate complex metabolic pathways in the postsynaptic cell to produce effects that cannot appropriately be called either excitatory or inhibitory (Squire & Kandel, 1999). This is particularly true of norepinephrine (noradrenaline), which, depending on specific circuitry and receptors, can mediate sympathetic arousal and/or agitation as well as parasympathetic calming. Thus, it is an oversimplification to rigidly call a neurotransmitter excitatory or inhibitory.

Transmitter Systems and Function

Neurotransmitters and their systems are often named for the receptors that they bind to (Schwartz, 1991).

Noradrenergic System

The noradrenergic system utilizes noradrenalin (also called norepinephrine) as its transmitter, which binds to noradrenergic receptors (on the ion channel) and often mediates either arousal or arousal regulatory mechanisms.

Dopaminergic System

The dopaminergic system utilizes dopamine as its transmitter, which binds to dopaminergic receptor sites and mediates aspects of motor function, reward, cognition, and endocrine mechanisms.

Serotonergic System

The serotonergic system utilizes serotonin as its transmitter, which binds to serotonergic receptor sites and mediates aspects of appetite, sleep, memory and learning, temperature, mood, behavior, muscle contraction, and the function of the cardiovascular and endocrine systems.

Glutamatergic System

The glutamatergic system utilizes glutamate as its transmitter, which binds to glutamatergic receptors and mediates at most synapses that are "modifiable," that is, capable of increasing or decreasing in strength. As we shall see at a later point, modifiable synapses are thought to be the main learning and memory storage elements in the brain (Kandel et al., 1991).

Cholinergic System

Finally, the cholinergic system utilizes acetylcholine as its transmitter, which binds to cholinergic receptor sites and mediates aspects of learning, short-term memory, arousal, REM sleep, and reward mechanisms.

Nontransmitter Chemical Signaling

Chemical signaling is not limited to synaptic transmitters or just to nerve cells of the brain. As multicellular organisms began to appear hundreds of millions of years ago, they evolved different tissue types that became specialized into different functional systems, such as the heart and the circulatory, gastric, and digestive systems. Consequently, two kinds of chemical signals evolved to coordinate the activities of the various tissues: *hormones* and synaptic transmitters (Squire & Kandel, 1999). Both forms of chemical communication have certain features in common.

Hormonal Transmission

In hormonal action, a gland cell releases a chemical messenger (a hormone) into the bloodstream to signal distant tissue. As an example, following a meal, the level of glucose (sugar) in the blood rises. This rise in glucose signals specific cells in the pancreas to release the hormone insulin, which acts on insulin receptors in muscle, so that glucose is taken up into muscle cells, then converted and stored as glycogen, the energy reserve form of glucose.

Differentiating Neurotransmitters and Hormones

There are, however, two major differences between hormones and synaptic transmitters. The first is that synaptic transmitters typically operate over much shorter distances than do hormones. Therefore, what makes synaptic transmission crucially different is that the membrane of the cell receiving the signal lies close to the cell releasing the signal. As a result, synaptic transmission is much faster than hormonal signaling and far more selective in its targets. The second difference between hormones and synaptic transmitters is that a single synaptic transmitter is able to produce a variety of different responses in target cells. By contrast, hormones tend to act over long distances throughout the body and always in the same way on a given set of target cells (Schwartz, 1991).

Electrical Potentials

Returning to our two electrical potentials, the synaptic potential and action potential are both electrical signals. However, the two differ markedly. Whereas the action potential is typically a large signal of about 110 mV, the synaptic potential is a much smaller signal, generating from a fraction of a millivolt to several tens of millivolts. This is dependent on a number of factors, which include the number of presynaptic terminals that are active and have, therefore, released neurotransmitters that reach the same postsynaptic cell (Squire & Kandel, 1999).

Synaptic Potentials

As was mentioned above, synaptic potentials are produced by the release of neurotransmitters from the vesicles (quanta), each of which is referred to as a miniature potential (Llinas, 2001). Basically, the resultant partial depolarization of the postsynaptic cell is referred to as a *synaptic potential*. This is the electrical signal that impacts the dendrites of the postsynaptic cell. These are considered local electrical events that can trigger chain-reaction events (other action potentials in the postsynaptic cell). However, although synaptic potentials are individually small, they can add together to create larger potentials. If there are enough of these events (incoming action potentials from other neurons) within a short time period, they may add up to partially depolarize the receiving cell to approximately –55 mV, leading to a full depolarization (+20 mV), creating another action potential (Llinas, 2001).

Comparison of Action and Synaptic Potentials

As was noted above, the action potential is all or none, whereas the synaptic potential is graded in strength. Finally, the action potential propagates actively and without fail from one end of the neuron to the other.

In contrast, the synaptic potential propagates passively and dies out unless it triggers an action potential in the postsynaptic cell. Therefore, the action potential carries the signal internally from one end of the cell to the other. In contrast, the synaptic potential mediates the movement of the signal from the postsynaptic terminals of the presynaptic cell to the presynaptic terminals of the postsynaptic cell, that is, from one cell (transmitting) to the other (receiving) (Llinas, 2001; Squire & Kandel, 1999).

Electrochemical Nature of Signaling

Hence, the transfer of signals from one neuron to another is first electrical (in the action potential), becomes chemical (in the synaptic transmission), and then becomes electrical again with the generation of the next action potential. Accordingly, neural communication is often referred to as "electrochemical coupling" or "electrochemical signaling."

Electrical/Electronic Synapses and Neural Synchronization

In contrast to the chemical synapse, where the space between neurons (the synaptic cleft) is in the order of approximately 20 nm, neurons forming electrotonic connections come into much closer contact (approximately 3.5 nm) and generate structural bridges between themselves. These electrically conductive bridges are called gap junctions (Bennett, 1997; Kandel et al., 1991).

Gap Junctions

At such junctions between two or more neurons, there are gap junction channels. If one injects fluorescent dye into one of these connected neurons, the flow of dye is unimpeded through these channels and, therefore, between all the cells connected (see Figure 3.3).

These gap junction channels allow conduction of ions (electrical current) directly between the cells, thus making them electrically coupled (Kandel et al., 1991). There are no neurotransmitters utilized in electrotonic flow, resulting in minimal, if any, delay in the voltage shifts created by the flow of electricity (ions) from one cell to another.

Comparing Gap Junctions and Chemical Synapses

In contrast, inherent in the process of electrochemical signaling is a small delay due to the many steps involved in the release of neurotransmitters,

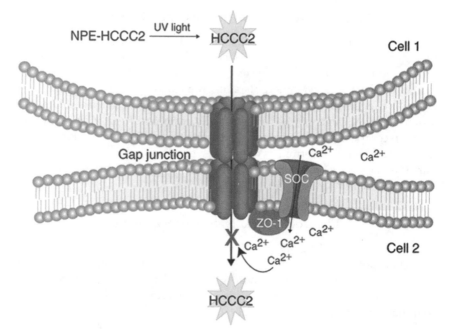

FIGURE 3.3   Diagram of a gap junction illustrating its function as a structural bridge, or tunnel, connecting one cell to the other.
Adapted from Spray, D.C. (2005). Illuminating gap junctions. *Nature Methods, 2* (1), p.13, with permission, Copyright 2005. Nature Publishing Group.

the diffusion time across the cleft, the subsequent transmitter binding, and finally, the activation of the respective ion channels to allow current flow in and out of the local area of the membrane. This process can take anywhere from 1 to 5 ms (Kandel et al., 1991; Llinas, 2001). On the other hand, with electrotonic connectivity, the ion flow is through channels that are already open, and current flows between cells directly, given that the interiors of the cells are interconnected. Consequently, when one neuron fires an action potential, any neurons that are electronically coupled to it are compelled to receive the signal simultaneously and fire to their action potentials.

Directionality of Ionic Gap Junction Flow

In addition, many gap junctions regulate ion flow in an even and *bidirectional* manner. This is in contrast to synaptic junctions, which allow ion flow in only one direction. This direct flow of current from neuron to neuron by means of electronic coupling results in rapid and synchronous firings of interconnected cells.

Neural Purpose of Gap Junctions

Why do we need electrical synapses? The main reason is that electrical synapses are not restricted to connections between two cells. Rather, they are found mostly in interconnected groups of similar neurons, where they serve to synchronize their activity. When several neurons are electrically coupled to one another, their ability to generate action potentials becomes elevated. In this way, groups of electrically coupled neurons are synchronized and become as one (Kandel et al., 1991).

Let us look at a simple example. Individual cardiac/heart cells can be experimentally grown in a special dish and, if kept separate, they will beat/contract on their own. These are the same cells as those that make up the two atria and two ventricles, the pumping chambers that cause the heart to contract. Once these single cardiac cells are allowed to come into contact with each other, they become electrotonically coupled, one cell to the other, whereupon they begin to beat together, as one. The larger the number of these cardiac cells, the faster it takes for their synchronization (Kojima, Kaneko, & Yasuda, 2004). Given that the function of cardiac cells is mechanical (to make the heart contract and pump), we can, therefore, state in mechanistic terms that the coordination/synchronization of the bioelectrical properties of these single cells, when added together, generates a *system*; in this case, it is a cardiac (atrial and ventricular) system.

Neural System Synchronization

In exactly the same manner, throughout the brain, electrotonic coupling synchronizes the activity of vast numbers of similar neurons, creating visual (color, shape, depth, etc.), auditory, emotional, cognitive, somatosensory, associational, and temporal/memory systems. As we shall see later, all aspects of information processing are mediated by linkages and binding within these systems. Llinas (2001) notes that chemical and electrical synaptic transmissions are ". . . the basic coinage that binds the different cellular elements into single multi-cellular functional states" (p. 91). These "single multi-cellular functional states" are the neural elements and foundation of any experience of consciousness and its inherent information processing.

Neuronal Oscillation

Oscillation, in general, is a rhythmic back-and-forth fluctuation within any aspect of natural phenomena. Neurons in the nervous system are endowed with particular types of intrinsic electrical activity that imbue them with particular functional properties (Llinas, 2001). Because neurons are similar to batteries, such electrical activity is manifested by variations (oscillations) in the minute voltage across the neuron's membrane (Llinas, 1988).

Oscillatory Mechanisms

As was illustrated above with respect to changing membrane potentials, oscillations are the result of the *depolarizations* and *repolarizations* that are caused by the neuron's interaction with other neurons. Simply put, oscillations in voltage derive from the changes in neural activity, as the membrane potential moves from resting potential (–70 mV) to pre-action potential (–50 mV), to action potential (+20 mV), to refractory potential (–80 mV), and back to resting potential (–70 mV). These oscillations in voltage remain in the local vicinity of the neuron's body and dendrites and are measured in hertz (Hz).

Depending on the type of neuron, these frequencies range from less than 1 Hz to more than 40 Hz. Llinas (2001) notes that on these voltage ripples, and in particular, on their crests, much larger electrical events, known as action potentials, are evoked. These electrical firings are the powerful and far-reaching electrical signals that form the basis for neuron-to-neuron communication. What will become obvious, as this exploration continues, is that oscillatory electrical activity, in all of its complex permutations, is not only paramount in neuron-to-neuron communication or whole-system functioning but is the electrical glue that allows the brain to organize itself functionally.

Coherence and Rhythmicity

Neurons that display *rhythmic* oscillatory behavior entrain to each other, electrotonically, via their action potentials (Llinas, 2001), becoming distinct, functionally *coherent* systems (Singer, 1993, 2001). In other words, by firing their action potentials simultaneously (as a result of electrotonic coupling), their voltage oscillations (voltage changes reflecting the change from resting to action potentials) are synchronized, allowing them to become as one. The resulting, far-reaching consequence of this function is that of neuronal groups that oscillate in phase, thereby creating aspects (representations) of human perception and functioning as a result of their synchronized oscillations (Braitenberg, 1978; Edelman, 1987; Palm, 1990; Singer et al., 1997).

Oscillatory Coherent Systems

As we noted above, for example, cardiac neurons synchronize their oscillations, becoming a local system of neurons that cause the heart to contract (Kojima et al., 2004; Llinas, 2001). Hippocampal neurons synchronize their oscillations to perform their part in memorial functions (Montgomery & Buzaki, 2007). The same holds true for somatosensory (Steriade, Amzica, & Contreras, 1996; Murthy & Fetz, 1996); visual (Gray, 1994); motor (Kristeva–Feige, Feige, Makeig, Ross, & Elbert, 1993); auditory (Eggermont, 1992;

DeCharms & Merzenich, 1996; Joliot, Ribary, & Llinas, 1994); amygdaloid (Collins, Pelletier, & Paré, 2001); cortical (Vaadia et al., 1995); and association (Jeffrerys, Traub, & Whittington, 1996) neuronal systems, as they synchronize their oscillations, respectively, creating their specialized/function-specific fragments of our consciousness.

Frequencies of Oscillations

As was noted, these oscillations occur at different frequency ranges, in different brain areas, and have been related to particular functions (Basar, Basar–Eroglu, Karakas, & Schürmann, 2000; Fernandez et al., 1998).

Parietal and Temporal Lobe Systems

In the parietal and temporal cortices, neurons tend to comprise the following two networks: one network tends to oscillate in the delta range (0.1–3 Hz) and is related, functionally, to deep sleep, offline information processing, and aspects of immune functioning; the other, oscillating in the theta range (3–8 Hz), is related functionally to aspects of REM sleep, offline information processing, and mediation of memory functions (Basar, Basar-Eroglu, Karakas, & Schürmann, 2001; Klimesch, 1999).

Occipital Lobe Systems

In the occipital cortex, neurons tend to oscillate in the alpha range (8–12 Hz) and are related functionally to aspects of visual processing (Klimesch, 1999).

Parietal and Frontal Lobe Systems

In the parietal and frontal cortices, neurons tend to comprise the following three networks (Hari, Salmelin, Makela, Salenius, & Helle, 1997): one network tends to oscillate at the low beta range (12–15 Hz) and is related to aspects of focus and attention; the second network oscillates in the mid-beta range (15–18 Hz) and is related functionally to mental ability, association, focus, and alertness; the third network oscillates in the high beta range (above 18 Hz) and is related to full functional alertness.

Interlobe System

Throughout the brain, interneurons (neither sensory nor motor) oscillate in the gamma range (31–100 Hz). Predominantly, though, these neurons tend to oscillate at approximately 40 Hz and mediate the synchronization, resonance, and binding of the various neuronal systems, noted above (Collins et al., 2001; Montgomery & Buzsáki, 2007; Sederberg et al., 2007; Steriade et al., 1996). We examine this in broader detail below.

Oscillatory Systems and Consciousness

As we have already seen and will become more evident as the book progresses, the signaling capabilities of neurons mediate all aspects of our mental life, from sensory perception to control of movement, to the generation of thought, to memory, to the experience and expression of emotion. Understanding the signaling properties of neurons, therefore, is essential for understanding the creation of neural systems as well as their synchronized functioning, creating system networks, which form the biological basis of any aspect of consciousness and information processing.

CHAPTER 4

Models of Information Processing

FOUNDATIONS

Two neurobiological models of information processing are currently dominant on the consciousness landscape: the *parallel distributed processing/con-
nectionism* and the *thalamocortical–temporal binding* models. Both have been
thoroughly researched and reflect agreement, at least with regard to the core
level of each model. Where controversy or disagreements do exist is generally
with regard to their finer points and details. However, when viewed analyti-
cally, these models are seen to either complement each other or in the sense
of one model picking up where the other leaves off. Accordingly, Damasio
(1999) notes that all the neurophysiological details of these processes have
not as yet been worked out, but a general conceptual framework has been
established.

Descriptive and Functional Anatomy

At this point, it seems reasonable to inquire as to which parts of the brain are
necessary for the creation of mind/consciousness and which may not be. In
the past 20 years, a great deal of light has been shed in the area of neurobiology. Much of the research has focused on the components that mediate our
emotional state of mind as well as those for information processing. In particular, the interrelationship between the function of brainstem structures, the
amygdala, thalamus, left dorsolateral prefrontal cortex, sensory and motor
areas, association cortices, and the hippocampus has been articulated with
increasing clarity. In order to understand the role of these structures in information processing, a brief description of their functional characteristics is
required (see Figure 4.1).

Medulla Spinalis—The Spinal Cord

The entire spinal cord does not appear to be an essential component of consciousness. The complete loss of the spinal cord has been shown to result in
severe motor defects, profound loss of body sensations, and some disturbance of emotional function. However, as long as the vagus nerve, which
runs parallel to the spinal cord, is preserved, the pathways of cross-signaling
between the body and the brain remain intact to mediate the aspects of
consciousness that require bodily input (Damasio, 2010). As an example,

Christopher Reeve's mind survived his extensive spinal cord damage, as did his consciousness.

The Amygdala

The amygdala is an almond-shaped cluster of interconnected structures perched above the brainstem. It is composed of two structures nestled in the temporal lobe, within the right and left hemispheres. The corticomedial amygdala is connected primarily with the olfactory bulb, the hypothala-

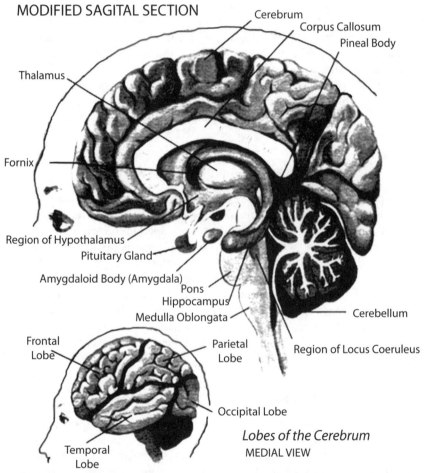

MODIFIED SAGITAL SECTION

Cerebrum
Corpus Callosum
Pineal Body
Thalamus
Fornix
Region of Hypothalamus
Pituitary Gland
Amygdaloid Body (Amygdala)
Pons
Hippocampus
Medulla Oblongata
Cerebellum
Frontal Lobe
Parietal Lobe
Region of Locus Coeruleus
Occipital Lobe
Temporal Lobe
Lobes of the Cerebrum
MEDIAL VIEW

FIGURE 4.1   Selected structures of the brain, ranging from the outer lobes to the innermost areas. Reprinted from *A Primer on the Complexities of Traumatic Memory of Childhood Sexual Abuse*, by Fay Honey Knopp & Anna Rose Benson, by permission of Safer Society Press.

mus, and the visceral nuclei of the brainstem. The basolateral amygdala is connected with the thalamus and parts of the cerebral cortex (Brodal, 1980, 1992).

The amygdala provides the central crossroads junction where information from all senses is tied together and endowed with emotional meaning. In the brain's architecture, the amygdala is poised like an alarm, wherein incomplete or confusing signals from the senses prompt the amygdala to scan experiences for danger. Sensory signals from the eyes, mouth, skin, and ears travel first in the brain to the thalamus and then across a single synapse to the amygdala. Sensory signals from the nose are routed directly to the amygdala, bypassing even the thalamus (LeDoux, 1986, 1992, 1994). A second signal from the thalamus is routed to the neocortex, the thinking brain. This branching allows the amygdala to respond before the neocortex, which mulls over information through several layers of brain circuits before it fully perceives and initiates a response (LeDoux, 1986).

Amygdaloid Activation

As the amygdala becomes aroused, from external stress, excitation, or internal anxiety, a nerve running from the brain to the adrenal gland triggers a secretion of epinephrine and, from the locus coeruleus in the brainstem, norepinephrine, both of which then surge through the body, eliciting alertness. These neurotransmitters activate the receptors on the vagus nerve (LeDoux, 1986). While the vagus nerve carries messages from the brain to regulate the heart, it also carries signals, triggered by epinephrine and norepinephrine, back into the brain. The amygdala is the main site in the brain where these signals are carried. They activate neurons within the amygdala to signal other brain regions to strengthen the memory of what just happened. This amygdaloid arousal seems to imprint in memory most moments of emotional arousal (pleasant or unpleasant) with an added degree of strength (Goleman, 1995). The more intense the amygdaloid arousal, the stronger the memorial imprint (LeDoux, 1986).

So, let us look at some examples of the amygdala's role in information processing. If I ask you (referring to residents of the United States, although it could pertain to citizens of other parts of the world) to tell me the date of President Eisenhower's death and where you were when you heard the news, I would guess that only some of you may remember the date and that very few of you, if any, will remember where you were when you received the news. On the other hand, if I ask the same question regarding President Kennedy's death, almost everyone in their late 50s or older will recall the date, where they were upon hearing the news, and possibly even the person delivering that news. For the younger readers, the same question could be applied to the terrorist attacks of September 11, 2001. The reason for the differences in information processing and memorial recall is the mediation of the amygdaloid system, which imbues the neural encoding of President Kennedy's death and

September 11 with profound emotion. Thus, to reiterate, the more intense the amygdaloid arousal, the stronger the memorial imprint.

The Dorsolateral Prefrontal Cortex

The brain's damper switch for the amygdala appears to lie at the other end of a major circuit to the neocortex, in the left prefrontal lobe, just behind the forehead (Brodal, 1980). Some of this circuitry is also found in the temporal lobe. This dorsolateral prefrontal part of the brain brings a more analytic and appropriate response to our emotional impulses, modulating the amygdala and other limbic areas (LeDoux, 1986).

This circuitry allows us to translate our *emotions*, which are physiological and visceral, into cognitive images/maps, which we call *feelings*; this allows us to understand and express that we are happy, sad, or angry. Although in normal parlance, the tendency is to refer to feelings and emotions interchangeably, they are nonetheless distinctly different phenomena from a neurological perspective, as they create completely different neural maps (LeDoux, 1996, 2002).

The presence of circuits, as noted above, connecting the amygdala to the prefrontal lobes implies that the signals of emotion, anxiety, anger, and terror, generated in the amygdala, can cause decreased activation in the dorsolateral area, sabotaging the ability of the prefrontal lobe to maintain working memory and homeostasis (Selemon, Goldmanrakic, & Tamminga, 1995).

The Hippocampus

The hippocampus has been referred to as the "gateway" to the limbic system (Winson, 1985). Like the amygdala, it is composed of two hippocampal structures, one in each of the hemispheres, adjacent to the respective amygdalae (Brodal, 1980, 1992). It is here that information from the neocortex is processed and transmitted to the limbic system, where memory and emotion are integrated (Reiser, 1994).

Accordingly, it appears to process memory in terms of perceptual patterns and contexts (LeDoux, 1992; van der Kolk, 1994). It is the hippocampus that recognizes the difference in significance of a bear that you see in the zoo versus one that you see in your backyard (Goleman, 1995). It also differentiates the significance of events that happened long ago from that of events that are recent (Reiser, 1994; Winson, 1985).

Bessel van der Kolk (1994) notes that when people are under severe stress, they secrete endogenous stress hormones that affect the strength of memory consolidation. He posits that "massive secretion of neurohormones at the time of the trauma plays a role in the long-term potentiation (and thus the overconsolidation) of traumatic memories" (p. 259). He cites LeDoux's (1986, 1992, 1994) work in noting that this phenomenon is largely mediated by the input of norepinephrine to the amygdala. This excessive stimulation of the amygdala interferes with hippocampal functioning, inhibiting cognitive evaluation of experience and semantic representation. Memories are then stored in sensorimotor modalities, somatic sensations, and visual images (van der Kolk & van der Hart, 1989).

Hippocampal Temporal Mediation

Let us look at an example of hippocampal temporal mediation of memory. Two Vietnam combat veterans are having a conversation. One of them has posttraumatic stress disorder (PTSD), whereas the other does not. Suddenly, a group of helicopters appears overhead. Given that helicopters were so prominent in the fighting in Vietnam, we can expect to see the following: The veteran without PTSD will be reminded of Vietnam and may shudder momentarily, saying, "Wow, that really took me back there, for a moment!" The veteran with PTSD will likely be triggered and become fearful of an impending attack.

So, why the difference? In the case of the veteran without PTSD, the experience of momentarily going back in time is quickly remedied by the hippocampal function (temporal memorial mediation) that differentiates past from present. The traumatized combat veteran, in the absence of temporal memorial mediation, will be unable to differentiate the past from the present, consequently finding himself, experientially, back in Vietnam.

Hippocampal Contextual Mediation

In the absence of hippocampal contextual mediation, traumatized people often are unable to differentiate dangerous situations from nondangerous ones (i.e., is the bear in the book, or in my backyard?). Consequently, they either perceive danger where there is none or are unable to identify danger when it is present, often putting themselves in harm's way.

In addition, the hippocampal neuronal network mediates the creation of a set of neurological "pointers," or links, to the information mediated by the other neural systems, when that information is needed for memorial recall (McClelland, McNaughton, & O'Reilly, 1995). This will be illustrated in detail below, as will the relationship of this function to thalamic binding.

The Association Areas

The associational cortices comprise most of the cerebral surface of the human brain and are largely responsible for the multifaceted (multimodal) processing that goes on *between* the arrival of input in the primary sensory cortices and the generation of behavior and/or thought. The varied functions of the association cortices are loosely referred to as "cognition," which speaks to the process by which we come to know the world. More specifically, cognition refers to *perception*, the capacity to attend to external stimuli or internal motivation *(sensation)*, to identify the significance of such stimuli, and to plan meaningful responses to them. Given the complexity of these functions, it is not surprising that the association cortices receive and integrate information from a variety of sources and that they influence a broad range of cortical and subcortical targets (Kandel, 1991a).

Inputs to the association cortices include projections from the primary and secondary sensory and motor cortices, the thalamus, and the brainstem. Outputs from the association cortices reach the hippocampus, the basal ganglia and cerebellum, the thalamus, and other association cortices.

Studies of lesions, neuroimaging, and electrophysiological recordings indicate that, among other functions, the *parietal–temporal–occipital association cortex* is especially important for attending to complex stimuli in the external (sensory) and internal environment (taking us from sensation to perception to language), the *temporal–limbic association cortex* is especially important for identifying the nature and significance of such stimuli, and the *prefrontal association cortex* is especially important for cognitively planning appropriate behavioral responses to the stimuli (Kupfermann, 1991b).

The Thalamus

The thalamus has been described as the gateway to the cerebral cortex and, thus, to consciousness. Like many of the major brain structures, the thalamus is bilateral. The two almond-shaped thalami are comprised of about 50 groupings of nerve cells, neural tissue, and fibers, called nuclei. With the exception of olfaction (smell), which is projected first to the amygdala, all external sensory input is projected first to the thalamus.

In addition, the thalamus is reciprocally interconnected with the prefrontal cortex, the basal ganglia, the somatosensory cortex, the association areas, the auditory cortex, the visual cortex, the motor cortex, the cerebellum, the brainstem, and limbic structures. The thalamus is, therefore, a relay center for top-down and bottom-up information processing. Its binding functions are activated by attentional aspects of arousal, alertness, or interest. As was noted above, and will be shown in detail below, its ability to synchronize the various neural assemblies throughout the brain, each oscillating at its own signature frequency, into infinite coherent combinations of functional networks may render it the cornerstone of perceptual, cognitive, memorial, and somatosensory integration.

The Cerebellum

Located behind the upper brainstem, it has been noted that within the enlarged, multifolded cerebellum, the number of nerve cells apparently exceeds the population in the cerebral cortex (Noback & Demarest, 1981; Shepherd, 1983; Zagon, McLaughlin, & Smith, 1977), making it the largest structure in the human brain (Williams & Herrup, 1988).

The cerebellum and its tremendous number of neurons is coupled with a high input-to-output axon ratio of 40:1 (Carpenter, 1991) and is reciprocally interconnected to parts of the brainstem, limbic areas, cerebral cortex, and the frontal lobes (Brodal, 1980; Larsell & Jansen, 1972; Llinas & Sotelo, 1992). Such a ratio of afferentation (input) to efferentation (output), combined with its comprehensive interconnectivity, suggests information processing, integration (Courchesne & Allen, 1997), and the consideration of the cerebellum as an additional association area in the brain (Leiner, Leiner, & Dow, 1986, 1991). This is a far cry from the traditional view that cerebellar mediation is limited to voluntary muscular movement and balance.

Accordingly, evidence has emerged that the lateral cerebellum is strikingly activated when an individual performs information processing (Courchesne & Allen, 1997), semantic association (Peterson, Fox, Posner, Mintun, & Raichle, 1989), semantic memory (Andreasen et al., 1995), and working memory (Awh, Smith, & Jonides, 1995), as well as declarative and episodic memory tasks (Andreasen et al., 1995). Based on its physioanatomical position, which allows it to affect known attentional systems, it has been shown for the past decade that the cerebellum contributes to attention operations by allowing attention to be shifted rapidly, accurately, smoothly, and effortlessly (Akshoomoff & Courchesne, 1992, 1994; Courchesne et al., 1994; Courchesne & Allen, 1997). The importance of this will be illustrated below, with respect to the role of the cerebellum in the mediation of the neural mechanisms underlying eye movement desensitization and reprocessing treatment.

Brainstem Structures

The foregoing neural structures comprise the traditional view that consciousness is mediated solely by cortical and limbic areas. Recently, however, Jaak Panksepp (1998), Bjorn Merker (2007), and others have argued that the first manifestation of consciousness originates in the brainstem. Damasio (2010) muses wryly that "the idea that mind processing begins at brainstem level is so unconventional that it is not yet even unpopular" (p. 75).

Recall Eric Kandel's (2006) argument that for some, the neurobiology of mind is potentially more disturbing because it suggests that not only the body but also the mind and the specific molecules that underlie our highest mental processes, of consciousness of self and others and of the past and future, have evolved from our animal ancestors. It certainly begs the question as to how our consciousness can be solely mediated by cortical and limbic structures that are uniquely human. We return to this below.

Brainstem Nuclei

Damasio (2010) argues that two brainstem nuclei, the nucleus tractus solitarius and the parabrachial nucleus, are involved in generating basic aspects of consciousness, namely, the sensations of pain and pleasure. Damasio suggests that these emotions

> . . . are, in all likelihood, the primordial constituents of mind, based on direct signaling from the body proper . . . they are also primordial and indispensable components of the self and constitute the very first and inchoate revelation to the mind, that its organism is alive. (p. 76)

Damasio (2010) notes that the conventional position posits that the left and right insulas (cortical structures) mediate the primordial emotions of pain and pleasure, noting further that studies have shown that the total destruction of the insular cortices (from back to front and in both left and right hemispheres) does not result in complete abolition of pain or pleasure (Damasio, Eslinger, Damasio, van Hoesen, & Cornell, 1985). Accordingly, he asserts that the nucleus tractus solitarius and the parabrachial nucleus send their signals on to the insular cortex, via thalamic nuclei.

Consequently, Damasio (2010) and Merker (2007) maintain that the brainstem nuclei would mediate the basic level of emotion (pain and pleasure), whereas the insular cortices would provide a more differentiated/complex version of those emotions and would also be able to relay those emotions to other aspects of cognition mediated by activity elsewhere in the brain.

Evolutionary Implications

If we examine this from an evolutionary perspective, the evidence is compelling. The nucleus tractus solitarius and the parabrachial nucleus receive comprehensive signals related to the state of the internal milieu in the entire body (Damasio, 2010; Dodd & Role, 1991). The signals originate in the spinal cord, the trigeminal nucleus, and even areas in the brain whose neurons respond directly to molecules traveling in the bloodstream. These signals mediate a comprehensive image of the internal environment and viscera (bodily organs), an image that constitutes the primary component of our emotions.

Recall that we noted that emotions are somatic and visceral, as opposed to feelings, which are the cortical, cognitive translation of our emotions. In addition, these nuclei are also richly interconnected with the periaqueductal gray (PAG). Panksepp (1998), Merker (2007), and Damasio (2010) have noted that the PAG is a complex set of brainstem nuclei and is considered the instigator of a large array of emotional responses related to defense, aggression, and pain. Additionally, laughter, crying, disgust, and fear are all triggered from the PAG. Therefore, the basic wiring map of these regions qualifies them for an image-making role, and the images that these nuclei create are our emotions.

Damasio (2010) argues,

> Because these emotions are early and foundational steps in the construction of the mind and are critical for the maintenance of life, it makes good

engineering sense (by which I mean evolutionary sense) for the supportive machinery to be based on structures that are housed literally next door to those that regulate life. (p. 80)

Hydranencephaly

Perhaps the most compelling evidence of brainstem mediation of consciousness can be seen in cases of hydranencephaly, wherein children are born with intact brainstem structures but without their cerebral cortex, thalamus, and basal ganglia. This tragic condition is often due to a major stroke, occurring in utero, resulting in the profound damage and reabsorption of the cortex, leaving the skull cavity filled with cerebrospinal fluid.

According to the conventional view regarding the mediation of consciousness, these children should be vegetative. Yet, observations of these children have shown evidence to the contrary. They appear to be able to move their heads and eyes freely and display expressions of emotion on their faces. These children not only are awake and often alert but also show responsiveness to their surroundings in the form of emotional or orienting reactions to environmental events, most readily to sounds but also to salient visual stimuli. They express pleasure by smiling and laughing and aversion by "fussing," arching of the back, and crying (in many gradations), their faces being animated by these emotional states (Shewmon, Holmes, & Byrne, 1999; Merker, 2007).

Therefore, in the absence of sensory cortices, whatever these children see or hear is mediated in the brainstem. Jaak Panksepp (1998), Bjorn Merker (2007), and Antonio Damasio (2010) have argued that the superior colliculi, a brainstem region that is closely interrelated with the PAG and indirectly with the nucleus tractus solitarius and parabrachial nucleus, is the candidate for such mediation. Consequently, Damasio suggests, whatever these children feel must therefore be mediated subcortically by the nucleus tractus solitarius and parabrachial nucleus, which are intact.

Primary Versus Reflective Consciousness

Reflection on the foregoing begs a number of questions. Why does the conventional view of consciousness negate the importance of brainstem structures? How important is it for us to appreciate the nuances of brainstem involvement in consciousness, given that we already have a clear picture of the sophisticated thalamocortical circuitry that mediates the complexity of our consciousness?

With respect to levels of consciousness, there is considerable agreement that a clear distinction exists between *reflective* and *primary* consciousness (Block, 2005; Chalmers, 1996; Edelman, 2006; Morin, 2006; Rosenthal, 2002). Reflective consciousness is characterized by symbolic processes, memory, and ultimately, the capacity for awareness of self and others and for monitoring one's own behavior. On the other hand, Merker (2007) and Panksepp

(1998) have argued that primary consciousness is *reflexive*, characterized by sensory processes that generate subjective experiences, such as emotions, and the awareness of and responsiveness to objects in the environment. Consequently, there is disagreement as to allowing both levels of consciousness to be considered. Many neuroscientists insist on limiting the definition to the inclusion of only reflective consciousness, arguing that anything less is not uniquely human but also indicative of other animal species. The opposing position has been elegantly articulated by Panksepp (cf. Merker):

> Consciousness is not critically related to being smart; it is not just clever information processing. Consciousness is the experience of body and world, without necessarily understanding what one is experiencing. Primary phenomenal states have two distinct but highly interactive branches: the ability to perceive and orient in the world; and the ability to feel the biological values of existence. . .if we wish to scientifically understand the nature of consciousness, we must study the sub-cortical terrain, where incredibly robust emotional and perceptual homologies exist in all mammalian species. Without work on animal models of consciousness, little progress, aside from the harvesting of correlates, can be made on this topic of ultimate concern. (p. 102)

This underscores a belief by many neuroscience investigators that a true understanding of human consciousness can be achieved only by relating human mechanisms of consciousness and information processing to the mechanisms of consciousness in other animal species. As was noted and will be examined in more detail, by studying habituation and sensitization in the mollusk Aplysia, the neural patterns of learning and memory were clearly and consistently codified for the first time. This research guided later studies of human memory and earned Eric Kandel the Nobel Prize in Physiology or Medicine in 2000. Although obviously to a more complex degree, what was learned from the nervous system of the Aplysia was found to be true in humans.

Implications for Medical Practice

Finally, on a less esoteric and more practical level, there are also ethical issues involved that relate to medical practice. From an ontogenic perspective (in utero development), the subcortical/brainstem capacity for consciousness, as noted above, appears to be present at approximately 30 weeks (Clancy, 1998; Myers & Bulich, 2005). Therefore, if we accept that a subcortical consciousness is possible by 30 weeks, then it would also appear more than possible that fetuses and neonates could experience something *approximating* pain.

Human neonates, preterm and full term, were thought to be insensitive to pain and were routinely subjected to surgical operations without adequate anesthesia or analgesia (Anand & Aynsley–Green, 1985; Anand & Carr, 1989). Large numbers of newborn infants are currently exposed to painful invasive procedures without appropriate analgesia (Johnston, Collinge, Henderson, & Anand, 1997; Porter & Anand, 1998; Simons et al., 2003) while recent medical reviews continue to question the ability of premature newborns or fetuses to experience pain (Derbyshire, 2006; Lee, Ralston, Drey, Partridge, & Rosen, 2005; Mellor, Diesch, Gunn, & Bennet, 2005).

Despite a higher prevalence of pain in patients with impaired cortical function (Breau, Camfield, McGrath, & Finley, 2004; Ferrell, Ferrel, & Rivera, 1995; Parmelee, 1996; Stallard, Williams, Lenton, & Velleman 2001), such patients, not unlike the children with hydranencephaly described by Merker (2007), receive fewer analgesics as compared with matched cognitively intact patients (Bell, 1997; Feldt, Ryden, & Miles, 1998; Koh, Fanurik, Harrison, Schmitz, & Norvell, 2004; Malviya et al., 2001; Stallard et al., 2001). Geriatric patients with dementia also receive fewer and lower doses of opioid or non-opioid analgesics than those received by comparable but cognitively intact older adults (Bell, 1997; Closs, Barr, & Briggs, 2004; Feldt et al., 1998; Forster, Pardiwala, & Calthorpe, 2000; Horgas & Tsai, 1998). Such is the folly of ignoring brainstem function in consciousness.

Parallel Distributed Processing/Connectionism

Parallel distributed processing (PDP) provides a framework for understanding the nature and organization of sensation, perception, thought, learning, memory, language, emotion, and motricity (motor function). According to the PDP model (McClelland, 1994; Rumelhart & McClelland, 1986), the mind is composed of a great number of unimodal (visual, auditory, olfactory, and tactile) and multimodal (perceptual, associational, somatosensory, emotional, and memorial) elementary units connected in neural networks or systems. The processing of information takes place through the interaction of these processing units, which are organized into modules. Therefore, mental processes (perception, learning, memory, cognition, emotion, language, and somatosensory integration) are interactions between these units/systems, which excite and inhibit each other in parallel rather than sequential operations. Accordingly, the active neural representation of information takes the form of a pattern of activation (a neural map) with respect to the units (unimodal and multimodal) that are, at any moment, involved in the processing of that specific piece of information. We will return to this in increasing detail.

Storage of Memory

In this context, knowledge or memory can no longer be thought of as stored in localized brain structures. Instead, it consists of and is stored as changes in synaptic strength between groups of units or systems that are distributed throughout the brain (Rumelhart & McClelland, 1986).

So, let us return to the example regarding the knowledge/memory that President Kennedy was assassinated on November 22, 1963. This type of knowledge or memory is stored as connection weights/synaptic patterns of strength between neural systems. When we think explicitly about our perception, knowledge, or memory regarding President Kennedy's death, we hold it in mind as a neural pattern (a map) of activation. Therefore, when we think about specific episodic memories, for example, we reinstate the pattern of activation (the neural map) representing the sensory aspects as well as the contextual elements, such as association, other memories, and emotion, that were involved in the encoding of this information.

Consequently, when people in their late 50s or older recall the date of President Kennedy's death, they not only recall it semantically (as a memorized or remembered historical fact), but many will also recall the day it happened, where they were when they heard the news, as well as their emotional reactions. So again, such memories are patterns of activation when we recall them, but the knowledge that allows this recall is stored in neural maps or engrams, which code the connection weights of these patterns of activation. Hence, memory is essentially the recreation of the neural map pattern (connection weights) that was created during the encoding of that information. Ostensibly, then, memories are not nouns but, rather, verbs (A. Konkle, personal communication, April 2009). Much more on this will follow, in layered detail.

Origins of PDP and Connectionist Theories

The ideas behind the PDP and connectionism approaches have a history that stretches back to luminous and insightful speculations originally articulated toward the end of the 19th century. It would not be until the 1960s that research techniques and designs would be available for the testing and proof of these brilliant speculative theories.

John Hughlings Jackson

Some of the earliest roots of these approaches can be found in the work of the neurologist John Hughlings Jackson (1869/1958), particularly in his persuasive criticism of the simplistic *localizationalist doctrines*, which promoted, for example, the notion that information processing was carried out by specialized cells in specific locations (i.e., memories were stored in memory cells). Jackson argued convincingly for distributed, multilevel conceptions of processing systems.

Sigmund Freud

Although not published in German until 1950 or translated into English until 1954, Sigmund Freud's *Project for a Scientific Psychology*, written in 1895, outlined a number of prescient ideas regarding learning and memory. Freud argued that the neural systems mediating perception differed with respect to neural plasticity from the neural systems mediating memory. Accordingly, Freud argued that the neural circuits mediating perception were seen to form synaptic connections that were rather fixed, thus ensuring the accuracy of our perceptual world. The neural circuits mediating memory were seen to form synaptic connections that change in strength with learning. Consequently, this neuroplastic mechanism was hypothesized to form the basis of memory and higher functions. We will return to this work further on in this text.

Santiago Ramon y Cajal

In a remarkable insight, Santiago Ramon y Cajal (1899), in addition to the seminal contributions noted above, formulated the synaptic plasticity hypothesis, which articulated the following: the strength of synaptic connections is not fixed but plastic and modifiable; changes in synaptic strength can be modified by neural activity such as perception; learning produces prolonged changes in the strength of synaptic connections by causing a growth of new synaptic processes; the persistence of these synaptic anatomical changes can serve as the mechanism for memory; neurons should be able to modulate their ability to communicate with one another; and the persistence of these alterations in basic synaptic communication, a functional property called synaptic plasticity, might provide the elementary mechanisms for memory storage. The testing and proof of these hypotheses would wait 75 years.

Donald Hebb

Equally insightful, Donald Hebb's (1949) formulations foreshadowed our state-of-the-art conceptualizations and understanding of cognition, memory, and consciousness in general. His conceptualizations of the "Hebb synapse" articulated that conditioned learning and memory were the result of changes in synaptic strength. His articulation of the "cell assembly" described organization among assemblies of cells, mediated by their intrinsic properties and hypersynchrony of neural firing. Regarding memory, Hebb postulated that when a neural assembly was firing as a result of sensory input, its activity represented the perception of the stimulus. When it fired in the absence of the corresponding sensory input, the activity represented the concept of the stimulus. As will become evident below, the similarity between this conceptualization and our current understanding of the relationship between perceptual encoding and memory recall is remarkable. He also noted that "any two cells or systems of cells that are repeatedly active, at the same time, will tend to become 'associated' so that activity in one facilitates activity in the other" (p. 70). This observation, often summarized by others as "neurons that fire together wire together," foreshadowed our understanding of neuronal assembly dynamics, state-dependent memory, and memory triggers.

Karl Lashley

A contemporary of Hebb, Karl Lashley (1950) also insisted upon the idea of distributed neural representation, echoing Jackson's criticism of the simplistic localizationalist doctrines. His insights into the function and storage of neural "engrams" were significant, and his essential understanding of distributed representation is captured in his insistence that,

> . . . the alternative to the theory of the preservation of memories by some local synaptic change is the postulate that the neurons are somehow sensitized to react to patterns or combinations of excitation. It is only by such permutations that the limited number of neurons can produce the variety of functions that they carry out. . . All of the cells of the brain are constantly active and are participating by a sort of algebraic summation in every activity. There are no special cells reserved for special memories. (p. 500)

The notion of algebraic summation foreshadowed the discovery of neural map summation (detailed below) that is inherent in thalamocortical–temporal binding. Similarly insightful was his awareness that memories are not stored locally in the brain but are distributed in fragmentary form and stored in neural maps (engrams).

Parallel Processing and Neuroplasticity

As we can see, it was already apparent in those early years of neural investigation and theorizing that the truly vast number of possible representations (sensory, perceptual, cognitive, memorial, somatosensory, motoric, linguistic, and emotional) that the brain needed to create at any given moment greatly exceeded the number of available neurons if these representations were to be solely mediated by specialized cells. What were needed were models of *neuroplasticity* that allowed for neurons to hold membership, interchangeably, in overlapping multiple assemblies. This would permit, for example, neurons to belong to assemblies that mediated arm position at one moment, velocity of movement at another moment, and hand gripping force a moment later. Only in this manner, distributed and parallel in function, could merely 100 billion neurons carry out their function in all aspects of consciousness.

The late 1960s and 1970s ushered in mathematical models (Anderson, 1973, 1977; Grossberg, 1976; McClelland, 1979; von der Malsburg, 1973; Willshaw, 1981) that attempted to codify further the existence of parallel distributed information processing.

Similar models under different names were also proposed as functional neuroimaging emerged. The transfer-appropriate processing model stated that memories are represented in terms of the cognitive operations that were engaged when the event was initially processed (Morris, Bransford, & Franks, 1977). Successful memory retrieval occurs when those earlier operations are recreated. In a similar vein, the cortical reinstatement model posited that the memory/recollection of an event occurs when a pattern of cortical activity/linkages corresponding to the encoding of the event is reinstated by activation of a hippocampally mediated recreation/relinking of that pattern (Alvarez & Squire, 1994).

Neural Mapping

In order to appreciate the *linkage* function of PDP and the *synchronization* role of thalamocortical–temporal binding, the process of neural mapping must be illustrated. The process of PDP creates neural *spatial maps*, whereas temporal binding creates neural *temporal maps* (Llinas, 2001). Put another way, spatial maps are maps of linked systems (oscillating at their own signature frequencies) that must be synchronized with respect to frequency, temporally (in real time), thereby creating temporal maps.

Although the management of life is unquestionably the primary function of human brains, it is hardly their most distinctive feature. There is certainly vast evidence that life can be managed without a nervous system, let alone a full-fledged brain. Many primitive life forms manage it, even unicellular organisms.

Mapping and Images

The distinguishing feature of brains such as ours is their uncanny ability to create maps. Neural mapping is vital for sophisticated information processing. Damasio (2010) argues that when the brain makes maps, it *informs* itself. The information contained in these maps can be used unconsciously to guide motor function and consciously to mediate sensation and perception. These functions pertain to most life forms. However, Damasio argues that "when brains make maps, they are also creating *images* [emphasis added], the main currency of our minds. Ultimately, consciousness allows us to experience maps as images, to manipulate those images and to apply reasoning to them" (p. 63). Therefore, the images resulting from neural mapping are visual, auditory, tactile, somatosensory, cognitive, associational, emotional, and memorial. They can also be beyond conscious awareness, mediating much of our motor function as well as aspects of our intrapsychic and interpersonal function.

The Structure of Maps

So, what exactly is a neural map? If you recall, we noted that neurons that display rhythmic oscillatory behavior entrain to each other, electrotonically, via their action potentials, becoming distinct, functionally coherent assemblies

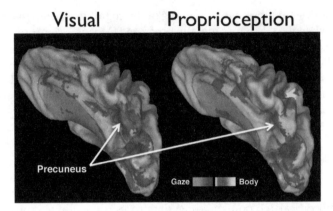

FIGURE 4.2   Brain maps above are represented by variations in shading. Visually-defined targets of reach are defined by a gaze-centered map. Reach directed toward unseen body locations, using the proprioceptive sense, uses a mental body map.
Pierre-Michel Bernier, UCSB Brain Imaging Center

and systems. Therefore, the consequences of this function are that of neuronal systems that oscillate in phase, thereby creating aspects (representations) of human perception and functioning.

The neural map is, essentially, another way of describing the linking (which creates spatial maps) and synchronized binding (which creates temporal maps) of these neural systems.

Neural Hardwiring Versus Neuroplasticity

Information processing goes beyond the brain's rigid *hardwiring*, which is reserved for neural regions, whose job it is to regulate the life process and which contain *preset maps* that represent varied aspects of our body and, therefore, cannot change their representation or mapping. This is because only a narrow range of body states is compatible with life and that we as organisms are genetically designed to maintain that narrow range and equipped to seek it, no matter what. The stability of that narrow range is mediated by the brain through an intricate neural programming and apparatus designed to sense minimal variations in the parameters of the body's physiological profile and to mediate the actions that correct those variations. There is no room for anything but minimal neural plasticity in these domains (Damasio, 1999, 2010).

Recall Freud's (1895/1954) visionary hypothesis regarding differences in systemic neural plasticity, wherein he posits,

> It would seem, therefore, that neurones must be both *influenced* [emphasis added] and also *unaltered, unprejudiced* [emphasis added] . . . the situation is accordingly saved by contributing the characteristic of being permanently influenced by excitation to one class of neurones, and, on the other hand,

that of unalterability . . . to another class. Thus, has arisen the current distinction between perceptual cells and mnemic cells. (p. 299)

Freud, in 1895, is proposing that the neural circuits mediating external sensory perception form synaptic connections (neural maps) that are rather fixed, thus ensuring the accuracy of our perceptual world. On the other hand, the neural circuits mediating learning and memory (referred to by Freud as mnemic cells) form synaptic connections (maps) that change in strength with learning.

Therefore, excluding the processes that regulate life (our physical plant) and external perception, our brain is constantly rewiring itself, expressing its neural plasticity, in reaction to our outer (sensory input) and inner (memory, associations and emotions) realities as different systems link and relink in infinite combinations and at lightning speeds. Accordingly, Damasio (2010) observes that, excluding basic physiology, brain maps are not static like classical cartography. Rather, he describes them as "mercurial, changing from moment to moment to reflect the changes that are happening in the neurons that feed them, which in turn reflect changes in the interior of our body and the world around us" (p. 66). Each wiring and rewiring creates its own neural map.

Recall Ramon y Cajal's (1899) prescient synaptic plasticity hypothesis, which articulated that the strength of synaptic connections is not fixed but plastic and modifiable and that changes in synaptic strength can be modified by neural activity such as perception and learning. As an illustration, let us return to President Kennedy's death. When Americans heard of the assassination, they processed this news perceptually, cognitively, somatosensorially, and emotionally. Therefore, their brains encoded this information via the parallel activation of visual, auditory, cognitive, associational, somatosensory, memorial, and emotional systems. These activations manifested in continuous changes in neural wiring and, therefore, synaptic strength, as people continued to experience the days that followed. Changes in synaptic strength are essentially changes in neural maps. As will be shown, these neural maps can now be visualized through the use of recent high-resolution multivariate analyses of functional magnetic resonance imaging (fMRI) and magnetoencephalography (MEG) data.

Mapping the Self and the Object

Neural maps are constructed as a result of our interaction with objects in the outside world. The term *interaction* is central, in that the making of neural maps, which is essential for motor function, often occurs in a setting of action to begin with. Action and neural maps, movements and mind, are essential parts of a continual cycle, a notion brilliantly described by Rodolfo Llinas (2001), who attributes the origin of the mind to the evolutionary necessity of the brain's control of organized movement. We will revisit this in detail below.

Maps are also constructed when we recall objects from the inside of our brain's memory banks or when we experience emotions. Damasio (2010) opines that construction of maps never stops, even in our sleep, as dreams demonstrate. He offers further,

> The human brain maps whatever objects sit outside it, whatever action occurs outside it, and all the relationships that objects and actions assume in time and place, relative to each other and to the mother-ship known as the organism . . . (p. 64)

Accordingly, consciousness, neural linkage, and neural mapping must be understood in terms of two key players, the *organism/self* and the *object*, and in the relationship that these players engage in over the course of their interactions. Damasio (1999) describes this elegantly, noting,

> The organism in question is that within which consciousness occurs; the object in question is any object that gets to be known in the consciousness process; and the relationship between organism and object are the contents of the knowledge we call consciousness. Seen from this perspective, consciousness consists of constructing knowledge about two facts: that the organism is involved in relating to some object, and that the object in the relation causes a change in the organism. (p. 20)

Hence, understanding the biology of consciousness becomes a matter of discovering how the brain is able to map the organism/self and the object and their neural impact on each other.

Temporal Binding

As we have seen, thus far, neural functions like perception, memory, language, and other aspects of consciousness are based on a highly distributed information processing system throughout the brain. One of the major questions, as yet, is how this information is synchronously integrated and how coherent representational states can be established in the distributed neuronal systems that subserve these functions. In other words, PDP and connectionism informs us of the construction and spatial mapping of the contents of these distributed neural systems. Therefore, PDP mediates the activation of the required systems (spatial maps) to be linked for any aspect of information processing. How, then, do these systems, each created by the synchronization of action potentials, each oscillating at their own signature frequency, bind together to form coherent and integrated perceptual, memorial, somatosensory, or emotional images and experiences (temporal maps)? So, if PDP supplies the parts/systems to be connected, as well as the spatial map to their locations, what is it that facilitates the connection/binding required for coherent and integrated (as opposed to fragmented) function and experience (temporal maps)?

These were the questions that were posed as the PDP and connectionism models were developed in the 1970s and 1980s and were referred to as the "binding problem." The 1980s also ushered in the use of magnetoencephalography, a technology that added magnetic resonance resolution to electroencephalography, thus facilitating the examination of neural network and system activation throughout the entire brain, simultaneously, in real time. The body of research that followed (to be detailed later) gave us the temporal binding model, that is, how many spatial maps (oscillating at their own signature frequencies) are synchronized and bound into one temporal map (oscillating at one network frequency).

Thalamocortical–Temporal Binding

Before we explore neural temporal binding, let us look at another example of a binding problem, one that was faced by musicians centuries ago, when they began to play in ensembles. In order for an ensemble to sound properly, the instruments must be in tune, simultaneously. In order to attempt such a tuning, the entire ensemble must play the same note. For instance, for concert bands and wind ensembles, the note/frequency of B flat is utilized and when sounded by the entire ensemble is referred to as a concert B flat. Typically, a wind ensemble is composed of brass, woodwind, and percussion instruments, as well as the conductor.

Those of you who are musicians know very well that if everyone in the band played the note B flat simultaneously on their instruments, the result would be a terrible cacophony of sound. Each instrument would produce the frequency of B flat. However, owing to the differing physics of these various instruments, their frequency modulation would not be synchronized, resulting in an awful noise. So, there must be a system that would allow for the appropriate modulation (or manipulation) of frequencies in each group (or system) of instruments, allowing them to synchronize their frequency output temporally (in real time), thereby producing the coherent sound of a concert B flat. The binding factor, in this case, is the conductor and his knowledge of the *theory of musical transposition*, which informs the practice of ensemble frequency modulation, based on the knowledge of the physical properties of the various instruments.

Accordingly, the conductor will suggest the following frequency modulations: the tubas, bassoons, oboes, and flutes will play B flat; the trumpets, trombones, tenor saxophones, bass clarinets, and clarinets will play C; alto and baritone saxophones and contrabass clarinets will play G; and the French horns will play F. When everyone in the wind ensemble plays the notes that they were instructed to play (i.e., modulate their frequencies), the result will be the temporally coherent sound of a concert B flat. Thereby, various systems of instruments (string, brass, and woodwind) oscillating at different frequencies are synchronized and bound to produce the coherent and unified phenomenon of one network frequency. As we shall see, the same process occurs in the brain.

The Binding Problem

Moving from musical ensembles to neural ensembles, we note similar problems. Given that sensory inputs generate but a fractured representation of our conscious experience (spatial maps), the issue of perceptual unity concerns the mechanisms that allow these different sensory components to be gathered into one global image or experience (temporal map). In recent years, this has been described as "binding", a process that is implemented by temporal conjunction, wherein simultaneous, real-time synchronization of various neuronal systems takes place (Bienenstock & von der Malsburg, 1986; Llinas, 1988; Gray & Singer, 1989; Singer, 1993; Llinas & Ribary, 2001). This dynamic interaction of neuronal assemblies/systems, based on temporal coherence (synchronization in real time), appears to generate flexibly dissipative functional neural structures (maps) capable of change as rapid as the perceptions they generate. These give the brain the ability to constantly, and flexibly, remap and reconfigure its neural assemblies, as needed.

Therefore, the principal assumption in this discussion is that the intrinsic electrical properties of neurons, and the dynamic events resulting from their connectivity, result in global resonant states, which we experience as integrated perception, cognition, and memory. Put another way, temporal binding is mediated by thalamocortical circuitry (detailed below), which binds coherently different neural systems (visual, auditory, tactile, somatosensory, olfactory, motoric, associational, memorial, linguistic, and emotional), each created by the synchronization of action potentials, each oscillating at their own signature frequency, to form coherent and integrated perceptual, memorial, somatosensory, or emotional images and experiences. Put yet another way, in addition to building complex maps in a variety of separate neural locations, the brain must relate the maps to one another, in coherent ensembles and in real time (Damasio, 2010). More on this later.

Forty-Hertz Gamma-Band Activity

As we have already seen, neural assemblies and systems are created by electrotonic/gap junctions and the resultant synchronization of action potentials. Consequently, each assembly and system resonates at its own common frequency. These frequency oscillations occur within different frequency ranges in different brain areas and have been related to particular neural functions. So, it should come as no surprise that cortical oscillations can also rally systems of neurons in widely dispersed regions of the brain to engage in coordinated and synchronized activity, much as a conductor would summon up various sections of an orchestra. So, what pattern of electrical activity exists in the brain that can accomplish this, and at what specific frequency?

Gamma Waves

Recent research in neuroscience utilizing magnetoencephalography indicates that 40-Hz oscillatory activity, generated by thalamic and cortical interneurons, is prevalent throughout the activated mammalian central nervous system, thus displaying a high degree of spatial organization (Collins et al., 2001; Jeffreys et al., 1996; Joliot et al., 1994; Montgomery & Buzsaki, 2007; Steriade et al., 1996; Vaadia et al., 1995). Therefore, inhibitory interneurons, at various cortical levels and particularly those of the reticular thalamic nuclei, would be responsible for the synchronization of gamma oscillations in distant thalamic and cortical sites. In other words, waves of gamma-band oscillations (40 Hz) would move throughout the brain in response to the need to synchronize the systems/maps that are being created and are active at any given moment.

It has been suggested that this 40-Hz activity reflects the resonant properties of the thalamocortical system, which is itself endowed with intrinsic 40-Hz oscillatory activity, generated by reticular thalamic and cortical inhibitory interneurons. Consequently, the 40-Hz gamma-band oscillatory activity serves to mediate global temporal mapping, by *scanning* for, *targeting*, and *synchronizing* the activity of the various neuronal assemblies and systems, each oscillating at its own respective frequency (spatial maps), creating network resonance, and binding them into a coherent and integrated outer and/or inner perceptual consciousness (temporal map) (Llinas, Leznick, & Urbano, 2003; Steriade, CurroDossi, & Contreras, 1993). We will consider this in further detail.

CHAPTER 5

Consciousness

PROCESSING OUR OUTER AND INNER REALITIES

Understanding consciousness and information processing, as we observed earlier, involves the solving of two interrelated problems. The first is the problem of appreciating how the brain, within the *self*, engenders the mental patterns and neural maps that generate the images, or representations, of an *object* (Damasio, 1999). These images can be sensory, tactile, cognitive, somatosensorial, associational, or emotional. Accordingly, such images can convey aspects of the physical traits of the object, reactions of like or dislike, one's plans for it, or its relationship to other objects. The second problem involves the understanding of how, in parallel with generating the mental patterns/maps of the object, "the brain also engenders a sense of self in the act of knowing" (p. 9).

So, how exactly does this look and feel? At this present moment, you are visualizing this page, reading the text, and constructing the meaning of my writing. The sensory images that you perceive externally as well as the related internal images you might recall might take up most of the extent of your mind but certainly not all of it. In addition to all the images, there is also the presence that represents you in a particular relationship with the object (my writing). Damasio (1999) asks, "If there were no such presence, how would your thoughts belong to you?" He offers,

> The simplest form of such a presence is also an image, actually the kind of image that constitutes a feeling. From that perspective, the presence of you is the feeling of what happens when your being is modified by the acts of apprehending something. The presence never quits, from the moment of awakening to the moment sleep begins. The presence must be there or there is no you. (p. 10)

Parallel Distributed Processing and Motor Function

Rodolfo Llinas (2001) argues that "the central generation of movement and the generation of mindedness are deeply related; they are in effect different parts of the same process. In my view, from its very evolutionary inception, *mindedness is the internalization of movement* [emphasis added]" (p. 5). Indeed, for Llinas, the mind is that class of all functional brain states in which *sensorimotor images*, including self-awareness, are generated. From this perspective, all neural images are considered sensorimotor in origin and constitute the conjunction or binding of all relevant sensory input (internal and external) to produce a discrete functional state that ultimately results in *action*.

Evolution of the Nervous System

Why is that, you might ask? To answer this question, one must ask another question: How and why did the nervous system evolve? Consequently, the first concern is whether a nervous system is actually necessary for all living organisms. The answer appears to be that it is not. Living *sessile* (lacking the capacity for movement) organisms, such as barnacles, coral polyps, or plants, have evolved quite effectively without a nervous system. Therein lies the first clue. The nervous system appears to be necessary only for creatures that express active movement, a biological property known as *motricity*.

Llinas (2001) notes that, interestingly, plants, which have well-organized circulatory systems but no hearts, appeared slightly later in evolution then did most primitive animals (with nervous systems). He argues that "it is as if sessile organisms had, in fact, chosen not to have a nervous system" (p. 15). What is clear, however, is that evolution chose to create organisms without a nervous system subsequent to its creation of organisms that did indeed possess nervous systems.

Motricity and the Brain

To illustrate the connection between the early evolutionary manifestations of a nervous system and the actively moving versus sessile (nonmoving) organisms, let us look at the primitive Ascidiacea, a sea squirt that represents an intriguing juncture in our own early chordate (true backbone) ancestry (cf Llinas, 2001).

The adult form of this creature is sessile, rooted by its pedicle to a fixed object in the sea. The sea squirt carries out two basic functions in its life. It feeds by filtering seawater, and it reproduces by budding. The larval structure, however, is briefly free swimming (usually for a day or so) and equipped with a brainlike ganglion containing approximately 300 cells.

This primitive nervous system receives sensory information about the neighboring environment through a statocyst (an organ of balance), a primitive light-sensitive patch of skin, and a notochord (a primitive spinal cord). These features enable this tadpole-like creature to react to and negotiate the ever-changing environment within which it swims. However, upon finding a suitable place in the sea, this tadpole-like larva proceeds to bury its head into the selected location, becoming sessile again. Once reattached to this stationary object, the larva absorbs and literally digests most of its own brain, including its notochord. It also digests its tail and tail musculature, thereupon reverting to the primitive adult stage, sessile and lacking a true nervous system, other than that required for activation of the simple filtering activity. Llinas (2001) opines that the lesson here is quite clear: The evolutionary development of a nervous system is an exclusive requirement and therefore a property of actively moving creatures.

Neural Automation and Fixed Action Patterns

Although the self is the centralization of prediction and action, it cannot orchestrate consciously every action that the body must accomplish from moment to moment, in a constantly changing external and internal world. Consequently, it utilizes a system referred to as *fixed action patterns* (FAPs) by Llinas (2001) and neural *dispositions* by Damasio (2010). These FAPs and dispositions comprise a set of well-defined neural motor patterns, that is, ostensibly ready-made motor maps. When switched on, these FAPs produce well-defined and coordinated movements, such as the escape responses (fight or flight), walking, swallowing, and other aspects of premotor and motor function. These FAPs and dispositions also mediate nonmotor functions, such as memory, emotion, and language, which we will explore later.

Accordingly, these neural patterns are seen to be "fixed" in that they appear to be stereotyped and relatively unchanging, not only individually but also in all individuals within a species. This fixedness can be observed from simple spinal reflexes (which do not require the brain) to complex motor patterns. For example, our walking, once initiated by the brain's upper motor system, with minor adjustments to the terrain, is mediated largely by circuitry in the spinal cord. The neuronal networks that mediate these specific stereotypical, often rhythmic and relatively unchanging movements are known as *central pattern generators*. These central pattern generators generate the neuronal patterns (rigid neural maps) of activity that drive the overt FAPs, such as walking.

Hence, FAPs can be seen as modules of motor activity that free the self from needlessly spending time and attention on every aspect of an ongoing movement or, indeed, on the movement at all. As a result, we may benefit from the experience of having walked for miles on a wooded path, almost blindly, while engrossed in a wonderful conversation with a friend. Consequently, if we recall this event, what may tend to come to mind most is the experience of our friend and our conversation. Our visual memory, however, may contain only details that drew our attention away from our friend or from the conversation, such as an event (e.g., stumbling) or the occurrence of something unusual in the setting. Otherwise, this walking FAP liberates us to spend time and attention on aspects of the experience that are more important than just managing our gait. Conversely, if we had to focus on every muscle and joint and the mechanics, consciously willing our basic locomotion, we could never enjoy the experience. Therefore, FAPs allow us the time and ability to multiprocess while mediating our motor activity in the background of our consciousness.

Frequent Action Patterns and Evolution

From the perspective of evolution and natural selection, one may wonder how an animal is able to implement particular desires or goals, given that these goals are often potentially executable in a staggering number of ways. Obviously, making the correct motor choice is fundamental to survival. Therefore, one may suspect that, at the very least, evolution and natural selection have somehow finely polished and ingrained into the nervous system mechanisms for the reduction of possible bad choices, which could be fatal errors. Accordingly, evolution and natural selection have done this, and these mechanisms are part of FAPs. Consequently, the nervous system's enormous number of degrees of freedom, or choices, is reduced by FAPs in the service of accurate prediction. At the same time, the ability to break or modify these constraining mechanisms, that is, the ability to override and make a choice, remains intact in humans.

Parallel Distributed Processing, Sensation, and Perception

Take a moment and look up from the page, noticing intently whatever is in front of you. Now, return to the page. In doing this, the many areas of your visual system, from the retinas to several regions of your cerebral cortex, shifted rapidly from mapping the book's page to mapping the room in front of you, then back to mapping the page again. If you now turn to the side and notice what is there, the mapping of the page ceases so that your visual–perceptual system can now map whatever you are seeing to the side. Ostensibly, then, in swift succession, precisely the same brain regions constructed a number of completely different maps by virtue of the different motor actions that you carried out. So, how does this happen?

Sensation

Information from the external world passes first through specific unimodal sensory (visual, auditory, motor, somatosensory, and olfactory) cortices that create separate internal representations/images of the observed stimulus in each sensory modality. These inputs are each processed by their respective regions of the unimodal sensory cortex (Lyons, Sanabria, Vatakis, & Spence, 2006; Macaluso & Driver, 2005; Martin, 1991; Squire & Kandel, 1999). As will be illustrated in detail later in this chapter, these sensory representations are then mapped and synchronously combined as a result of the mediation of the thalamus and the

thalamocortical neuronal network circuitry (Llinas, Grace, & Yarom, 1991; Llinas & Ribary, 2001; Singer, 1993; Steriade, Jones, & Llinas, 1990).

Perception

By this time, some conscious but incomplete perception or trace of the sensations has occurred (Schacter, Chiu, & Ochsner, 1993). As this information
flows through the perceptual representation system, a memory of the sensation is formed within it (Squire & Kandel, 1999). From the sensory cortices,
information flows into other neural networks. One set of pathways carries
information to regions of the association cortex where multimodal representations (perceptual, associational, linguistic, emotional, and memorial) are con-
structed/mapped (Macaluso & Driver, 2005; Martin, 1991; Squire & Kandel,
1999).

For visual perception, information is transmitted to the parietal–temporal–
occipital association cortex, where the object is identified and, through the
mediation of language areas, is named (Ishai, Ungerleider, Martin, Schouten,
& Haxby, 1999). The identification of sounds heard or objects touched is mediated by similar pathways. In order for stable memories to form, the neuronal
network of the hippocampal complex is required. Simultaneously, information from both perceptual and semantic representational networks flows into
the hippocampal complex.

Hippocampal Mapping

The hippocampal network mediates two major functions (McClelland et al.,
1995). Initially, while the memory traces formed in the perceptual and semantic memory networks in the cortex are too weak to support direct recall, the
hippocampal neuronal network mediates the formation of a stable memory,
combined with the associated affect (emotional content or valence) mediated
by the amygdaloid neuronal network, resulting in the capacity of long-term
recall. However, memories are not stored in the hippocampus. For that matter, as we observed, there appear to be no memory centers, or memory neurons, where complete memories are stored (Squire & Kandel, 1999).

Accordingly, the hippocampal neuronal network mediates the creation
of a set of neurological "pointers" or links to the information mediated by the
other neural systems (McClelland et al., 1995). These pointers include links
to all sensory modalities that were activated during the event, any semantic
memories initially activated by the sensory input, material processed by the
association area networks, and the emotional responses to it, mediated by the
neuronal activation of the amygdaloid neuronal network (McClelland et al.,
1995; Nadel & Moscovitch, 1998; Squire & Kandel, 1999; Stickgold, 2002). The
total of synchronized activations of neuronal networks (spatial maps; each
oscillating at their own signature frequencies) that were required to encode/

create a "unified" perception (temporal map) is referred to as an *engram* (Squire & Kandel, 1999).

Engrams

Damasio (2010) notes that these mapped patterns, or engrams,

> . . . constitute what we, conscious creatures, have come to know as, sounds, touches, smells, tastes, pains, pleasures, and the like—in brief, images. The images in our minds are the brain's momentary maps of everything and of anything, inside our body and around it, concrete as well as abstract, actual or previously recorded in memory. (p. 70)

Accordingly, the words in this text that are being utilized to convey these ideas to you were initially formed in my mind as auditory, visual, or somato-sensory images prior to my implementation of them into their written version. Similarly, you initially process these written words as verbal images (visual images of written language) before their actions on the brain promote the evocation of yet other images of a nonverbal kind. These nonverbal images allow you to mentally process the concepts that correspond to these words.

In addition, any feelings or associations in the background constitute mapped images, as well. Damasio (2010) argues that at the highest level of abstraction or introspection, these images probably result from the *brain's making maps of itself making maps*. At this level, images may find their way into musical compositions, literature, or abstract mathematics. Consequently, minds manifest in a flowing combination of actual images and recalled images, in an ever-changing matrix.

Finally, the images derived from sensation and perception can be either conscious or nonconscious. Images continue to be produced perceptually or from recollection, even in the absence of conscious awareness. Yet, in many instances, such images are capable of influencing our thoughts, emotions and, actions.

In summation, perceptual images are driven by changes that occur in the body and brain as a result of our interaction with the world (the object). Signals sent by sensors throughout the body organize neural patterns that map our interactions with the objects in our world. These neural patterns are formed fleetingly in the wide-ranging sensory and motor regions of the brain that normally receive signals from specific body regions. Therefore, brain mapping is the functional feature of a neural system dedicated to managing and controlling the life process.

At its simplest level, sensorial and perceptual mapping can detect the presence and position of an object in space or its trajectory. This enables us to track danger or an opportunity and to avoid it or seize it. At higher levels, when our minds avail themselves of sophisticated compound maps of every sensory variety and create a multifaceted film-like perspective of the world external to us, we can react to the object and events in that world with greater precision. Moreover, once maps are committed to memory and can be re-created in imaginative recall, we are enabled to plan ahead and engineer enhanced responses.

Parallel Distributed Processing and Memory

Recall some of your most vivid memories and notice the detail. The core element that renders these memories vivid will be their emotional saliency, in that the encoding of these experiences will certainly have taken place under circumstances that were either very pleasant or very unpleasant. Provided that a perceptual event has significant value and, therefore, emotion, the multimedia sights, sounds, touches, feels, smells, and such will be brought back, on cue.

Consider now the wonder that is memorial recall and reflect on the resources the brain must have to construct it. Beyond perceptual images in diverse sensory domains, the brain must have the means of storing the particular neural patterns and must maintain a pathway to retrieve the patterns for the attempted reproduction/recall to work. Once all of this is accomplished, we experience the *phenomenon* of recalling something. Our ability to negotiate the complex world around us is solely dependent on this ability to learn and recall. Damasio (2010) argues that "our ability to imagine possible events also depends on learning and recall and is the foundation of reasoning and navigating the future and, more generally, for creating novel solutions for a problem" (p. 131).

Hence, a number of questions come to mind. What precisely changes in the brain when we learn and then remember? Do declarative and nondeclarative memory employ different brain systems and utilize different strategies for storing memory? Do these distinct memory systems make use of different molecular steps for storage, or are the storage mechanisms essentially similar? How does short-term storage vary from long-term storage? Do they occur at different neural locations, or can the same neurons store information from both short- and long-term memory?

Classifying Memory

Some uncertainty still exists about precisely how many discrete memory systems there are and how they should be named. Nonetheless, a general agreement has emerged about the foremost memory systems and about the brain areas that are most essential for each memory system.

Declarative Memory

Declarative memory mediates the recall of facts, ideas, and events, that is, for information that can be brought to conscious recollection as a verbal proposition or as a visual image. This type of memory has also been referred to as *explicit* or *episodic*.

Another type of declarative memory, originally described in 1972 by Endel Tulving, is referred to as *semantic memory*. Rather than mediating the recall for specific facts or events, considered the domain of episodic memory, semantic memory mediates conceptual knowledge.

Episodic Versus Semantic Memory

Very little of what we have experienced is remembered as episodic memory. As an example, an average 40-year-old would have had approximately a quarter of 1 million hours of waking experience. However, such a person may not posses even 1,000 hours of memories recallable in the full detail of their original sensorimotor and emotional richness (Stickgold, 2002). Instead, their brain will have extracted, abstracted, and stored the critically useful information contained in all these hours of experience. So, for example, we may no longer retain the episodic memory regarding the day we learned how to add in arithmetic or who sat next to us. What we retain is the semantic memory and understanding of the additive function in arithmetic. Similarly, we retain the semantic memory for arithmetic subtraction and multiplication as well as the semantic memory for grammar and writing.

Semantic processing can also go beyond cognitive conceptual meaning. It can mediate the meaning or significance of events in our life. As an example, the positive cognitions utilized in EMDR can be seen as semantic processing. The semantic aspect of an event is often more important than the episodic/memorial aspect. Think of it: "It's over" can be more important than "it was awful and frightening and I thought that I was going to die." This is a deeper level of semantic processing.

Nondeclarative Memory

Nondeclarative memory also results from experience but is expressed as a change in behavior or emotion rather than as a recollection. Unlike declarative memory, nondeclarative memory is unconscious or implicit. When we learn motor skills, we refer to it as procedural memory. When it involves emotional learning, we refer to it as habituation, sensitization, or conditioning.

Early Research on Memory

In order to understand the complexity of learning and memory in the human brain, the progression of research studies, beginning with simple animals such as mollusks, needs to be examined, sequentially. Kandel (2006) opines,

It is an explicit hypothesis of this research that the potentiality for elementary forms of conditioned plastic change is an inherent and fundamental property of all central nervous collectivity, whether simple or complex . . . . I was testing the idea that the cellular mechanisms underlying learning and memory are likely to have been conserved through evolution and therefore to be found in simple animals, even when using artificial modes of stimulation. (p. 162)

Informed by Ramon y Cajal's (1899) *synaptic plasticity hypothesis*, the initial studies on learning and memory focused on habituation, sensitization, and classical conditioning, all forms of nondeclarative learning and memory.

Habituation

As a result of habituation, the simplest form of learning, an animal can learn to recognize the harmlessness of a stimulus. For example, when an animal perceives an unexpected noise, it initially responds with a number of defensive alterations in its autonomic nervous system, including dilation of the pupils and increased heart and respiratory rates. If the noise is repeated numerous times, the animal's pupils no longer dilate, and its heart and respiratory rate no longer increase. Through habituation, the animal has learned that the stimulus can be safely ignored. If the stimulus is removed for a time and then presented again, the animal will respond to it again. Such is the nature of short-term habituation.

Regarding evolution's design, the elimination of responses that fail to serve a functional purpose focuses an animal's behavior. Immature animals often show flight responses to an array of nonthreatening stimuli. Once they become habituated to such stimuli, they can focus on stimuli that are novel or associated with pleasure or danger. Accordingly, habituation, as a form of learning and memory, is important in organizing perception.

In humans, owing to its simplicity as a test for recognizing familiar objects, habituation is one of the most accurate means of studying the development of visual perception and memory in infants. Analogous to animals, infants typically respond to a novel image with dilated pupils and increased heart and respiratory rates. If shown an image repetitively, they will stop responding to it. Therefore, infants who have been repeatedly shown a circle will ignore it. However, if the infants are shown a square, their pupils will again dilate, and their heart and respiratory rates will increase, indicating that they can distinguish between and remember the two images (Kandel, 2006; Squire & Kandel, 1999). As we will see later, habituation is parasympathetic (neurally inhibitory and calming) in nature and geared toward orienting and information processing.

Sensitization

Sensitization can be seen as the mirror image of habituation. Rather than teaching an animal to ignore a stimulus, sensitization is a form of learning in that it teaches the animal to focus and respond more vigorously to almost any stimulus after having been exposed to a threatening stimulus. As an example, immediately after a shock has been applied to an animal's foot, the animal will consequently display exaggerated withdrawal and escape responses to a bell, a tone, or even a soft touch.

Like habituation, sensitization as a method of learning and memory is common in people. Accordingly, after hearing a gun go off, people will typically show an exaggerated response and will jump when they hear a tone or sense a touch on the shoulder. Sensitization heightens our responses, making us focus more intently, at times to the point of being anxious or even to the point of being traumatized. Consequently, as we will see later, in contrast to habituation, which is parasympathetic and geared toward information processing, sensitization is sympathetic (neurally excitatory and arousing) in nature and therefore geared toward action.

Classical Conditioning

Classical conditioning was first described by Ivan Pavlov (1927) at the turn of the 20th century. While studying the digestive reflexes of dogs, Pavlov discovered that a dog would start to salivate at the sight of an approaching attendant who had fed the dog in the past. Pavlov observed that an initially neutral, weak, or otherwise ineffective stimulus could become effective in producing a response as a result of having been associated with a strong stimulus. In this case, the research attendant was the initially ineffective or *conditioned stimulus*, and the attendant associated with or paired with the dog's food, the effective or *unconditioned stimulus*. After repeated pairing, Pavlov discovered that the conditioned stimulus (the attendant) was able to elicit salivation on its own. Pavlov referred to the salivation as the *conditioned response*.

With respect to learning, humans and simpler animals need to distinguish predictive relationships between events in their environment. They must be able to discriminate food that is edible from food that is sickening or poisonous and predator from prey. From an evolutionary perspective, humans and animals can obtain the appropriate knowledge in one of two ways: either innately, resulting from the hardwiring of the nervous system, or by learning through experience. In humans, a great deal of emotional learning takes place through this process. We will return to this.

Studies of Habituation

The first attempt at the neural analysis of habituation was undertaken as early as 1906 by Sir Charles Sherrington, focusing on a cat's limb withdrawal, involving a memory lasting a few seconds. In 1966, Thompson and Spencer attempted a similar study, finding that habituation led to a decrease in synaptic activity in the interneurons (neurons that are interposed between the sensory neurons that detect touch and the motor neurons that signal muscles to contract). However, the organization of neurons in the spinal cord proved too complex and difficult to examine. These and similar studies made it clear that scientists required simpler neural systems to study if they were to observe and analyze specific neural patterns and circuits. Consequently, a number of researchers turned to invertebrate animals such as snails and flies because their nervous systems contained a relatively small number of cells, rendering the process of cellular and neural analysis simplified and accurate.

Eric Kandel and his colleagues realized that the Aplysia, a large marine snail, was perfectly suited for studies of habituation and sensitization. The Aplysia has a defensive gill withdrawal reflex that is in some way comparable to the limb withdrawal reflex in the cat. When either the mantel shelf or the siphon is gently touched, the siphon contracts, and the gill withdraws rapidly and protectively into a cavity beneath the mantel shelf.

In their studies on habituation, Kandel and his colleagues (Thompson & Spencer, 1966; Kupfermann, Castellucci, Pinsker, & Kandel, 1970; Tigh & Leaton, 1976; Bailey & Chen, 1983) repeatedly applied a weak and harmless stimulus to the siphon. Typically, the experimenter would touch the siphon with a fine paintbrush, causing both siphon and gill to withdraw briskly. Utilizing different protocols, they were able to produce in the Aplysia short-term memory of 10 to 15 minutes' duration as well as long-term memory storage that lasted in excess of 3 weeks. The reader is referred to Squire and Kandel, 1999, and to Kandel, 2006, for further elaboration on these fascinating experimental procedures. So, what did these studies teach us?

Short-Term Habituation

The neural circuitry for this behavior by the Aplysia was delineated in the early 1970s by Kandel and his colleagues Irving Kupfermann, Vincent Castelucci, Jack Byrne, Tom Carew, and Robert Hawkins. With this knowledge, these researchers could now address the following question: How can learning occur and memory undergo storage in a prewired neural circuit? Kandel and his colleagues found the answer to be clear-cut. Although the pattern of connections of the gill withdrawal reflex is set once and for all early in development, the precise strength of the connections is not.

In other words, there is the existence of plasticity (the ability to modify and change). In response to a novel stimulus to the siphon, the sensory neurons receiving information from the siphon excited the interneurons and gill motor neurons rather vigorously. As this stimulus was repeated successively, the action potentials in the sensory neurons did not as readily produce an action potential in either the interneurons or the motor neurons. Whatever action potential was created to the latter stimuli was so weak as to trigger only a few and, finally, no resultant action potentials in the target motor neurons. The net result of this weakening in synaptic connections (relative to the initial control situation) was the learned and remembered (short-term) cessation of the gill withdrawal reflex.

With respect to short-term learning and memory, these studies confirmed Ramon y Cajal's (1899) prescient hypothesis that basic elementary synaptic connections undergo plastic change as a consequence of learning and that these changes are sufficiently consistent to form the cellular basis for short-term memory storage (Squire & Kandel, 1999; Kandel, 2006). In addition, the cause of the changes in synaptic strength was known to be the result of a change in the number of neurotransmitter vesicles released from those terminals. Recall from Chapter 3 that the coinage that regulates synaptic strength is neurotransmission. These studies also codified, for the first time, that memory storage, for even a simple nondeclarative memory, is distributed through multiple sites rather than located in one memorially specialized site.

In summary, Squire and Kandel (1999) argue that the major importance of these early studies is the illustration that,

> Nondeclarative memory storage does not depend on specialized memory neurons whose only function is to store information. Rather, the capability for simple nondeclarative memory storage is built directly into the synapses connecting the neurons that make up the neural circuit of the behavior being modified. Memory storage results from changes in neurons that are themselves components of the reflex pathway. (p. 42)

They are not specialized memorial circuits. In this respect, as we shall explore further, nondeclarative memory differs from declarative memory in that some specialized temporal lobe circuitry (the hippocampal formations) is required for storing the capacity to reactivate the respective neural patterns that mediate conscious recall. However, even in this case, the majority of the circuitry involved is, nonetheless, not memory-specialized and thus reflective of the neural patterns that were gleaned from the Aplysia's learning and memory.

Long-Term Habituation

We have thus far considered short-term memory. What about long-term memory? As we noted above, in contrast to the training toward short-term habituation, Kandel and his colleagues found that by utilizing four training sessions of 10 trials a day, spaced over 4 days, habituation (memory) that lasted in excess of 3 weeks was produced. The questions to be answered at this point were the following: How do the short- and long-term forms of memory relate to each other? Do they occur at different loci or at a common locus?

Accordingly, they tested the connections between the sensory neurons and motor neurons known to be involved in short-term habituation 1 day, 1 week, and 3 weeks after the training. They found a 60% decrease in the synaptic connections between sensory and motor neurons. Thus, whereas the short-term habituation involved the transient decrease in synaptic strength, long-term habituation produced the more prolonged change, a complete inactivation of many of the previously existing connections. In addition, the number of synaptic connections among sensory neurons and motor neurons decreased, signifying changes in the physical structure of the neuronal circuits.

These experiments illustrate a number of features of nondeclarative memory. First, the experiments offer direct evidence that just as short-term memory involves short-term changes in *synaptic strength*, long-term memory necessitates long-term changes in *synaptic strength and structure*. Second, the same elementary synaptic connections can participate in the storage of both short- and long-term memory. Third, not all synapses in Aplysia are plastic and adaptable, in that some synaptic connections in the nervous system do not change their strength.

However, as synapses that have evolved to participate in memory storage, a relatively small amount of learning produces large and enduring changes in synaptic strength that may persist for weeks. Finally, the results signify that synapses are plastic not only with respect to the amount of neurotransmitters that they release but also in their shape and structure. As we shall see later in this chapter, these changes in the physical structure of neurons represent the elementary anatomical basis for long-term memory storage in all species, including humans.

In the Aplysia, these simple memories are stored as a weakening of strength of preexisting synaptic connections. These findings, which emerged in the early 1970s, provided the initial evidence for Ramon y Cajal's (1899) suggestion that the persistence of alterations in basic synaptic communication, a functional property called synaptic plasticity, might provide the elementary mechanisms for memory storage.

Kandel (2006) notes that, most importantly, these studies illustrated that long-term memory was not merely an extension of short-term memory. In long-term memory, not only do the changes in synaptic strength last longer, but also, more astonishingly, the actual number of synapses in the circuit changes. Specifically, in long-term habituation, the number of presynaptic connections among sensory neurons and motor neurons decreases. This occurs in contrast to short-term habituation, wherein the changes are solely in the strength of the existing synapses. We shall return to this.

We have thus far examined only the simplest form of nondeclarative memory: the trace in the brain as an animal learns and remembers to ignore a stimulus. A number of questions come to mind: Do more complex forms of learning also institute memory traces by altering the strength of synaptic connections? If so, can connections be strengthened as well as weakened? What are the molecular mechanisms whereby synapses are altered in strength? Does learning enlist novel types of molecules that are dedicated for memory storage, or does memory borrow molecules used for other purposes?

Studies of Sensitization

Short-Term Sensitization

The initial clues to the molecular mechanisms of memorial processes emerged from the study of sensitization, a form of nondeclarative learning that results from an increase in synaptic strength. In contrast to habituation, wherein an animal learns about the characteristics of a benign or trivial stimulus, with sensitization, an animal learns about the properties of a harmful or threatening stimulus. Therefore, sensitization is a form of learned fear, in that it teaches the animal to focus and respond more vigorously to almost any stimulus after having been exposed to a noxious or threatening stimulus.

As we noted above, in contrast to habituation, which is parasympathetic and geared toward orienting and information processing, sensitization is sympathetic in nature and, therefore, geared toward the sharpening of our defensive reflexes, in preparation for fight, withdrawal, or escape (Squire & Kandel, 1999). We will return to this in detail, later in the book. Therefore, in the case of habituation, one has an altered response to a stimulus following recurring presentations of the same stimulus. In contrast, in the case of sensitization, one has an altered response to a stimulus as a consequence of exposure to some other, unusually noxious, stimulus.

As an example, we return again to the Aplysia, wherein the foundation of our current understanding was created. Kandel and his colleagues found that subsequent to the Aplysia receiving a shock to its tail, its reaction to siphon stimulation was substantially strengthened, in that it withdrew its gill more completely than it would under normal circumstances. The animal's memory for this noxious stimulus, as measured by the length of time it remembered to exaggerate its gill withdrawal reflex each time the siphon was touched, became more enduring the more often the noxious stimulus was repeated. Squire and Kandel (1999) note that a single shock to the tail produced a short-term memory that persisted for minutes. Four or five shocks produced a long-term memory that lasted for 2 or more days, and further training produced a memory that lasted for many weeks.

So, if habituation leads to a decrease in synaptic strength, does sensitization lead to an increase? Indeed, the studies on sensitization evidenced increases in synaptic strength in the networks of sensory neurons and interneurons impacting on motor neurons, when comparing postlearning to prelearning (Kandel, Brunelli, Byrne, & Castellucci, 1976; Bailey & Chen, 1983; Hawkins, Abrams, Carew, & Kandel, 1983). These were the same sets of synapses that had been depressed by habituation.

Taken together, these studies illustrated that, at different times, the same set of synaptic connections can be modulated in opposite directions by different forms of learning, and as a result, the identical set of connections can participate in mediating different memories. Therefore, synapses that increase in strength, at any given time, can serve as memorial mediation for certain kinds of learning, for example sensitization and classical conditioning. These are the same synapses that, at another time, decrease in strength to serve as a mediation process for other kinds of learning, for example, habituation. In habituation, we would say that the synapses have been *depressed*, whereas in sensitization, we would say that they have been *facilitated*.

Long-Term Sensitization

As we noted above, four or five shocks produced the long-term memory that lasted for 2 or more days, and further training produced the memory that lasted for many weeks. As in the habituation studies, the data illustrated again that long-term memory was not simply an extension of short-term memory. Accordingly, in the long-term habituation studies, the number of presynaptic connections among the sensory neurons and motor neurons decreased in number, whereas in long-term sensitization, sensory neurons grew connections that persisted as long as the memory was retained.

These anatomical changes were expressed in several ways. Kandel (2006) notes that in long-term sensitization, the number of presynaptic terminals more than doubles (from 1300 to 2700), increasing the proportion of active synapses from 40% to 60%. In addition, there was an outgrowth from the motor neurons to receive some of the new connections.

These studies provided the first clear evidence regarding the two competing theories of memory storage. Consistent with the *one-process* theory, the same neural site can mediate both short- and long-term memory in both habituation and sensitization. Furthermore, in each case (habituation and sensitization), changes in synaptic strength occurred. However, consistent with the *two-process* theory, the data showed clearly that the mechanisms of short- and long-term change were intrinsically different. Whereas short-term memory produced changes in the function of the synapses (strengthening or weakening preexisting connections), long-term memory necessitated anatomical changes. Hence, recurring sensitization training caused neurons to grow new terminals, giving rise to long-term memory, whereas habituation caused neurons to retract existing terminals. Consequently, by creating profound neural structural changes, learning could make inactive synapses active or active synapses inactive.

Classical Conditioning

In 1983, Kandel and his colleagues discovered that the gill withdrawal reflex of Aplysia could be classically conditioned (Carew, Hawkins, & Kandel, 1983). This finding in itself was extremely important, in that the data illustrated that even the simple reflex behavior in a relatively simple animal could be altered by associative learning, a process profoundly more complex than habituation and sensitization, which are nonassociative forms of learning.

In order to produce classical conditioning in Aplysia, a mild touch applied to the siphon was used as the conditioned stimulus, and a stronger electrical current applied to the tail was used as the unconditioned stimulus. When these two stimuli were paired for approximately 10 trials, the mild stimulation of the siphon alone was able to elicit the marked withdrawal of both the gill and the siphon. As was discovered in the habituation and sensitization studies, extended training (learning) led to the same progression, from short- to long-term memory.

So, what happens inside the nervous system to mediate this type of learning and memory? Kandel and his colleagues discovered that the sensory neurons release even more neurotransmitters as a result of conditioning than after sensitization. Therefore, at least in this part of the reflex, classical conditioning relies on the manifestation of the same mechanism that is utilized in sensitization. Squire and Kandel (1999) argue that the studies of classical conditioning make two vital points. First, they present yet another case of the many aspects of a single synapse, given that we see the same synaptic connections participating in still a third variety of learning and thereby contributing to still a different memory storage process. Second, they illustrate that even rather complex forms of learning and memory storage nonetheless utilize the same elementary mechanisms of synaptic plasticity, both pre- and postsynaptically, "in combination, almost like a cellular alphabet" (p. 64).

Long-Term Memory and Molecular Genetics

In order to understand the next phase of research by Kandel and his colleagues and, consequently, the underlying mechanisms of long-term and permanent synaptic changes and memory storage, a brief exploration of molecular genetics is required.

Classical *Mendelian genetics* and its current application to behavioral genetics describe the manner in which genes modulate behavior, psychological traits, and psychological experience. On the other hand, the question explored by modern *molecular genetics* is rather the opposite: How do the extrinsic sensory experiences of our outer environment and our intrinsic psychobiological experience of our inner environment modulate gene expression? The understanding that human experience at the level of information processing is so intimately associated with gene expression on a biological level is one of the most surprising findings of current research in molecular genetics.

Molecular Genetic Studies

In the late 1970s, as the structural/anatomical foundations of short- and long-term memory storage in Aplysia were becoming consistently clear, Kandel and his colleagues turned their attention to their molecular underpinnings. They discovered, in both short- and long-term memory storage, a cellular program of gene expression and resultant changes in molecular protein synthesis. Their findings illustrated consistently that short-term memory storage involved gene expression, resulting in the modification of preexisting proteins. This was expressed as a change in the effectiveness of preexisting synaptic connections.

In contrast, the long-term forms of memory storage required more complex gene expression and new protein synthesis and were expressed structurally by the growth and maintenance of new synaptic connections. Specifically, proteins known as *prions* were found consistently to act as a neural *self-perpetuating switch*, enabling the maintenance of long-term synaptic changes (neural maps/engrams), which remain stable, encrypted, and retrievable upon demand. Therefore, short-term memory storage was shown to be mediated by changes in the existing neural circuitry, whereas long-term memory storage required the growth of new circuits.

The articulation and explanation of the underlying molecular biology of the various gene expressions and protein syntheses is beyond the scope of this book. The reader is referred to Bailey, Bartsch, and Kandel (1996) and to Kandel (2006) regarding the elaboration of the mechanisms of cyclic adenosine monophosphate (cAMP), protein kinase A, cAMP-responsive element-binding protein, and cytoplasmic polyadenylation element-binding prion protein.

Kandel (2006) concludes that "thus in Aplysia, we could see for the first time that the number of synapses in the brain is not fixed—it changes with learning! Moreover, long-term memory persists far as long as the anatomical changes are maintained" (pp. 214–215). In other words, these studies identified, for the first time, the mechanisms underlying the creation, stabilization, and reactivation (memorial recall) of the Aplysia's neural maps. We would learn in the ensuing decades that this conclusion, articulated in the 1980s, would prove to be equally true when applied to the human brain and its elaboration of complex forms of memory.

Explicit Memory Research

In 1990, at the age of 60 years, emboldened by the recent development of methods for inserting and deactivating individual genes in mice, Kandel turned his attention to the hippocampus and explicit memory. Mice offered a superb genetic system for examining the role of individual genes and synaptic modification on the one hand and intact behavior, in the form of explicit memory storage, on the other. In addition, mice had well-developed medial temporal lobes and hippocampi, characteristics paramount for explicit memory.

Kandel realized that these advances in genetic engineering made the mouse a superb experimental animal for identifying the genes and proteins responsible for the various forms of long-term potentiation and its concomitant memory storage. One could then relate these genes and proteins to the storage of spatial memory. Although mice are relatively simple mammals in comparison to humans, they possess a brain that is anatomically similar to that of humans and, as in humans, the hippocampus is involved in storing memories of places and objects, that is, explicit memory.

In addition, techniques had become available for limiting the expression of newly implanted genes as well as for controlling the timing of gene expression in the brain, thereby making it possible to turn the gene on and off. Consequently, the effects of specific genes could now be studied by specifically activating or deactivating them.

Driven by his keen understanding of evolution, Kandel had always predicted that the basic underlying mechanisms of learning and memory in snails would have to be true (albeit more complex) with respect to humans. Nonetheless, this would of course have to be proven. The study of explicit spatial memory in mice would bring his research that much closer to human functioning.

In a series of ground-breaking papers, Kandel (1989, 1998, 2000) documented that *explicit* hippocampally mediated memory in the mammalian brain involved increased gene regulation. As in the Aplysia studies, the storage of long-term explicit memory also gave rise to anatomical changes, specifically the growth of new synaptic connections. Regarding evolution, Kandel (2006) noted that "despite the significant behavioral differences between implicit and explicit memory, aspects of implicit memory storage in invertebrates have been conserved over millions of years of evolutionary time in the mechanisms by which explicit memory is stored in vertebrates" (p. 294). These findings, in combination with the Aplysia studies as well as studies on other animals, made it clear that several key molecular mechanisms of memory are shared by all animals.

Neural Mapping Studies

As Kandel was pursuing these inquiries, the study of neural mapping was bringing forth increasing insights. In 1971, O'Keefe and Dostrovsky made a groundbreaking discovery regarding the hippocampus's processing of sensory information. They discovered that neurons in the hippocampus of the rat registered information that was not sensory but related to the space surrounding the animal.

They found that as the rat walked around an enclosure, some hippocampal pyramidal cells fired action potentials only when the animal moved into a particular location, whereas others fired action potentials when the animal moved to another place. As we now know to be true in humans, the rat's brain was breaking down its surroundings into many small, overlapping areas, similar to a mosaic, with each represented by activity in specific cells in the hippocampus. By studying the firing of hippocampal pyramidal cells, O'Keefe and Dostrovsky (1971) were able to verify that the hippocampus of a rat contained an inner representation, a *neural map*, of its external space.

Kandel understood that the study of explicit spatial memory, involving complex neural and especially hippocampal mapping, would create the next bridge to the understanding of human memory storage. With regard to spatial memory, the difference between mice and humans is not that significant. In all living creatures, from snails to humans, knowledge of space is of critical importance to behavior and all other aspects of consciousness. O'Keefe & Nadel (1978) argued that "space plays a role in all our behavior. We live in it, move through it, explore it, defend it" (p. 5).

Not surprisingly, Kandel and his colleagues discovered that some of the same molecular actions responsible for long-term potentiation were, indeed, necessary for preserving the spatial map over a long time. Blocking protein synthesis disrupted the neural map and the rats' ability to remember, giving clear direct genetic and structural evidence that the neural map correlated with and mediated explicit spatial memory. Specifically, more complex protein *prions* were again found consistently to act as a neural self-perpetuating switch, enabling the maintenance of long-term synaptic changes (neural maps/engrams), which remain stable, encrypted, and retrievable upon demand. This series of studies earned Kandel the Nobel Prize in Physiology or Medicine in 2000.

The Evolutionary Imperative

The reciprocally reinforcing results utilizing snails, flies, mice, and rats were profoundly reassuring. These were very different animals, examined for diverse types of learning and memory, which were studied utilizing profoundly dissimilar approaches. Jointly, they illustrated clearly that the cellular mechanisms underlying different forms of memory appeared to be the same in many animal species and for many different forms of learning because those mechanisms had been conserved through evolution.

In addition, these studies also reinforced another important biological principle: that evolution does not require new, specialized molecules to produce a new adaptive mechanism. It was already known at this time that nonneuronal systems such as the gastrointestinal, kidney, and liver utilized similar genetic messaging and protein synthesis. This was found even in the bacterium E. coli. Therefore, the biochemical actions underlying the mediation of learning and memory did not arise specifically to support memory. Rather, neurons simply recruited an efficient signaling system employed for other purposes in other cells and used it to produce the changes in synaptic strength required for memory storage.

Francois Jacob (1982) argued that evolution is a *tinkerer*. It uses the same collection of genes time and again in slightly different ways. It works by varying existing conditions, by sifting through random mutations in gene structure that give rise to slightly different variations of a protein or to variations in the way that protein is deployed in cells. Put another way, evolution as a tinkerer

> . . . manages with odds and ends . . . . uses whatever he finds around him, old cardboard, pieces of string, fragments of wood or metal, to make some kind of workable object. The tinkerer picks up an object that happens to be in his stock and gives it an unexpected function. Out of an old car wheel he will make a fan; from a broken table a parasol. (p. 35)

Kandel (2006), grounded by his keen understanding of evolution, was, throughout his career, assured that his findings would point the way to the substrates of human memory. Like Jacob, he understood that in living organisms, new capabilities are achieved simply by modifying existing molecules slightly and adjusting their interaction with other existing molecules. He noted,

> Because human mental processes have long been thought to be unique, some early students of the brain expected to find many new classes of proteins lurking in our gray matter. Instead, science has found surprisingly few proteins that are truly unique to the human brain and no signaling systems that are unique to it . . . . all life, including the substrate of our thoughts and memories, is composed of the same building blocks. (p. 236)

Human Long-Term Memory Storage

As we noted above, the complete neurophysiological details of these processes are not, as yet, known, but their broad contours are already understandable. What appears to be most evident is that memories consist of and are stored as changes in synaptic strength within assemblies of neurons (Squire & Kandel, 1999), which when activated *create the experience* of recalling a memory.

As we noted, there is no separate memory center where memories are permanently stored. A rather a long line of evidence (McClelland et al., 1995; Nadel & Moscovitch, 1998; Herrmann, Munk, & Engel, 2004; Slotnick, 2004; Prince, Daselaar, & Cabeza, 2005; Mulligan & Lozito, 2006; Osipova et al., 2006; Jokisch & Jensen, 2007; Montgomery & Buzsaki, 2007; Sederberg et al., 2007) indicates that memories appear to be stored in the same distributed assemblies of brain structures that were engaged in initially perceiving and processing what is yet to be remembered.

Therefore, the brain regions in the cortex that are involved in the perceiving and processing of color, size, shape, and the various other object attributes are close, if not identical, to the brain regions important for remembering. Ostensibly, remembering is the reactivation of the majority of the components (synchronized neuronal assemblies) of the engram or neural map that was used to encode the experience that one is trying to remember (Squire & Kandel, 1999).

Damasio (2010) notes that when we encode an encounter with any object (person, place, experience, etc.) in our environment, it is more than just its visual structure that is mapped in optical images of the retina. The following neural maps are also recorded: first, the sensorimotor pattern/map associated with viewing the object (such as eye and neck movements or entire body movements, if applicable); second, the sensorimotor pattern/map associated with either touching and/or manipulating the object, if applicable; third, the sensorimotor pattern/map resulting from the evocation of previously acquired associations and memories pertinent to the object; and fourth, the sensorimotor pattern/map related to the triggering of emotions and feelings relative to the object. Note that these neural maps are described as sensorimotor because we perceive by engagement with the object, not by passive receptivity.

Structure of Memory

What we generally refer to as the memory of something (the object) is actually the reactivation of the majority of the temporal maps/engrams, described in the paragraph above, that were activated during the encoding. Robert Stickgold (2002) describes this in another way, noting that "what occurs in reality when we *store a memory* [emphasis added] is that we simply alter a system so that a certain pattern of brain activity and hence perception or thought is more likely to be reinstated in the future" (p. 64). The memorial activation pattern is obviously not identical to that of the encoding pattern, in that the neural pattern of activation with respect to the eyes or ears, for example, would not be reactivated, because we would be *remembering*, not *experiencing*, an external event. On the other hand, the neural patterns (maps) created in the visual and auditory cortices would be reactivated because we would be experiencing an internal event known as memory. Therefore, memory is not a facsimile of something to be remembered, a sort of a hard copy stored in a file. As we noted above, it is not a noun but rather a verb, a recreation of what was once created.

Engrams and Neural Linkage

What is required to facilitate the reactivation of these engrams (spatial maps; i.e., to remember something) appears to be the activations of the hippocampus and other areas of the parahippocampal region. Therefore, the hippocampal formation serves an integrative function (McClelland, 1994, 1996; Squire & Kandel, 1999), linking together the various neuronal assemblies that were established independently, in several cortical regions throughout the brain, so that ultimately, these assemblies are again activated as a synchronized network (Montgomery & Buzsáki, 2007; Prince et al., 2005).

So, how is this linking of neural maps accomplished? Recall that we explored the brain's rigid hardwiring, which is reserved for neural regions whose job it is to regulate the life process and which contain *preset* maps that represent varied aspects of our body and other physiological parameters and, therefore, cannot change their representation or mapping. Memorial recall also requires preset maps but of a different nature.

Neural Dispositions

As we noted above, Damasio (2010) refers to these preset maps as *dispositions* and posits that for a long time in evolution, brains operated solely on the basis of these dispositions or Llinas's (2001) FAPs. However, as organisms became more complex and sophisticated, they developed the capacity for neural mapping that went beyond formulaic responses. Consequently, their responses became customized to objects and situations rather than being generic and instinctive, allowing for more precise and sophisticated function. Damasio argues,

> The fascinating fact, then, is that the brain did not discard its true and tried device (dispositions) in favor of the new invention (maps and their images). Nature kept both systems in operation and with a vengeance: it brought them together and made them work in synergy. As a result of the combination, the brain simply got richer, and that is the kind of brain we humans receive at birth. (p. 135)

As a result of this hybrid mixture of preset dispositions and plastic neural mapping, which we have inherited from many prior species, we are equipped with rich networks of dispositions that run our basic mechanisms of life management. They include, in addition to running our bodily physical plant, the nuclei that mediate our endocrine system, together with the nuclei that mediate the mechanisms of reward and punishment, the activation and linking of memorial maps, and the triggering and execution of our emotions. It is as a result of this combination of systems that emotions are expressed somatically and viscerally in the body. We will return to this in further detail.

Returning to memory, when human brains decided to create enormously large files of recorded images but lacked space to store them, they appear to have borrowed the dispositions approach to solve this engineering dilemma (Damasio, 2010). Given that it was not possible to store memories as microfilm or some other version of hard copies in files, nature appears to have evolved the hippocampus and surrounding hippocampal regions, allowing them to mediate memorial dispositions as a sort of formula for the reconstruction of neural maps, and utilized our existing perceptual machinery to reassemble them as best it could. That is why when we remember someone, for example, our perceptual system allows us to see and/or feel that person, so to speak, in our mind. Therefore, neural maps are recorded and stored in dispositional (unconscious/implicit, encrypted, and dormant) form: waiting to become activated conscious/explicit images, actions, or memories, on demand. Again, we see the tinkering of evolution at work.

Memorial Consolidation and Long-Term Potentiation

What are less clear are the processes of memorial consolidation, wherein episodic memory is eventually converted to semantic memory, and long-term potentiation, wherein the reconstruction of neural maps (required for memory) is enabled over the span of many decades.

Off-Line Memory Consolidation

Robert Stickgold (2008) opines,

> Memories are not like photographs. They evolve. After a memory is initially formed, it goes through an extended period of consolidation—a complex set of automatic processes, occurring without intent and outside of conscious awareness—that modifies the memory. (p. 289)

Consequently, a memory can be considerably different from its original structure, with some aspects as vivid as the day they were formed and others forgotten. Throughout this process, memories become integrated into a wide-ranging memory network, creating historical context for the original memory and, in the process, constructing an intrinsic, implicit (personal and subjective) interpretation of the event.

Sleep

During the past decade, a robust and rapidly growing literature has demonstrated that sleep plays a vital part in the innate, automatic, and unattended processing of memories, across days, months, and years. Specifically, this literature has illustrated consistently that sleep contributes to processes that change memories after they are formed (encoded), thereby strengthening, stabilizing, and integrating these episodic memories into general semantic memory networks. Recall that our brain will have extracted, abstracted, and stored the critically useful information contained in all our hours of experience.

Memory structures (neural maps) that are active during the encoding of experiences are, by and large, reactivated, at times with significant temporal precision, during subsequent sleep. This has been illustrated in studies of single neurons (Pavlides & Winson, 1989), neural networks in animals (Wilson & McNaughton, 1994), and whole-brain regions in humans (Peigneux et al., 2004). These findings support the hypothesis that reactivation of memories during sleep enhances the representation (neural maps) of such memories within the brain. Robert Stickgold (2007) argues that such enhancement can result from the following: strengthening the synaptic connections that were created during the encoding of the experience; creating similar neural connections to create alternative representations of the learned information in other brain regions; and connecting the recently learned memory to other related memories. Although the earlier studies noted above were co-relational by design (i.e., examining only whether the variables studied were related positively or negatively or were nonrelated), a number of recent studies have provided direct experimental support for these hypotheses.

Sleep and Insight

In an interesting study of sleep-dependent memory (Wagner, Gais, Haider, Verleger, & Born, 2004), subjects were taught a complex set of rules for solving a group of mathematical problems. Unbeknownst to the subjects, a simpler solution also existed that allowed the problem to be solved without any calculations. When the subjects were retested 12 hours after their initial training, a number of subjects discovered this simpler method of performing the task. However, the number of subjects gaining this insight more than doubled after a night of sleep. Consistent with older studies, this study illustrated that not all types of sleep are equally effective in facilitating this form of insight. Accordingly, the 60% of the subjects who gained this insight the next day evidenced significantly less non-REM sleep [also referred to as slow-wave sleep (SWS)] than the 40% who did not develop this insight.

Stickgold (2008) notes that in spite of the fact that neither REM sleep nor light non-REM sleep showed a significant increase, the decreased deep SWS suggests that it was REM sleep that was critically important. Therefore, the most remarkable finding of this study is that during sleep (markedly absent of deep non-REM SWS), the brain is able to analyze and manipulate information, gathered from early experiences, to facilitate the development of associations and ensuing insights during subsequent waking function, even when the individual is consciously unaware that there is any insight to discover.

This phenomenon is strikingly similar to our description of semantic processing, wherein information networks link to other *apparently* unrelated information networks to produce new insights. We will return to this phenomenon when we examine its similarity to EMDR processing and the tenets of the adaptive information processing (AIP) model.

Sleep and Episodic Memory

In a more recent study on episodic memory, Rasch, Buchel, Gais, and Born (2007) present compelling evidence that experimentally reactivating memories during sleep, on the night following learning, can enhance those memories. In this study, the authors used an unusually designed task, in which subjects were exposed to the scent of roses whenever they successfully matched a pair of cards while playing a memory game, similar to the game of concentration. Afterward, that night, when sleep recordings indicated that the subjects were in deep SWS, the subjects were again exposed to the rose fragrance.

The following morning, subjects exposed to the rose fragrance during sleep demonstrated superior memory for the location of the previously learned matched pairs. Even more important, Rasch et al. (2007) demonstrated by means of neuroimaging that spraying the rose scent during SWS also led to specific activations of the hippocampus, the area of the brain most implicated with the reactivation of neural maps/engrams during memorial recall. They argue that reactivating just this single contextual feature of the memory/neural map (the rose fragrance) caused the hippocampus to complete the episodic memory trace/neural map, reactivating the entire memory of the learning task and thereby facilitating its consolidation and enhancement.

With respect to the dynamics of long-term memory consolidation, the study also illustrated that one of its mechanisms appears to be sleep-mediated strengthening of neuronal maps and the concomitant stabilization, strengthening, and conversion of neural memorial maps into more permanently retrievable structures.

REM Versus Non-REM Sleep

These recent studies offer support to previous evidence that suggests that REM and non-REM sleep serve related but distinct functions in off-line memory processing, with non-REM sleep appearing most critical for strengthening of hippocampal episodic memories and REM sleep for the creation and strengthening of neocortical semantic memories (Plihal & Born, 1997).

Consistent with this, deep-brain studies of rats have shown that information flows out of the hippocampus and into the cortex during non-REM sleep (suggestive of the strengthening of hippocampally mediated episodic memory) and then reverses direction during REM sleep, flowing from the neocortex into the hippocampus (suggestive of the creation and strengthening of cortical and semantic memory; Buzsáki, 1996). It is likely, given what we have seen of evolution's consistency and only slight tinkering, that we will one day find a similar neural sleep pattern in humans.

Accordingly, studies have shown that in humans, REM sleep preferentially activates weak associations (indicative of semantic processing), but non-REM sleep activates strong associations (indicative of the strengthening of episodic memory (Stickgold, Scott, Rittenhouse, & Hobson, 1999). These data represent the contours of our understanding of off-line information processing, with the fine details yet to be inferred.

Long-Term Potentiation of Human Memory

Recall that studies of snails, flies, mice, and rats have illustrated that in contrast to short-term memory, long-term memory (i.e., the ability to retain information for several hours, days, and decades) depends on the expression of genes and the consequent protein synthesis that give rise to stable and retrievable anatomical changes (neural maps). Specifically, proteins known as *prions* have been found consistently to act as a neural self-perpetuating switch, enabling the maintenance of long-term synaptic changes (neural maps/engrams), which remain stable and retrievable upon demand.

Given the complexity of the human nervous system, the definitive exploration of the underlying molecular biology of long-term memory has for the most part eluded us. However, bearing in mind the lessons learned from evolution's steady but ever-so-slight tinkering, it has long been suspected that the basic molecular mechanisms found consistently in snails, flies, mice, and rats must also be found, at least in basic form, in humans. Not surprisingly, then, Papassotiropoulos et al. (2005), scientists at the University of Zurich, found that the *prion protein* gene (PRNP) plays a key role in human long-term memory by mediating (as in mollusks, flies, rats, and mice) a neural self-perpetuating state that facilitates the maintenance of long-term synaptic changes (neural maps/engrams), which remain stable and retrievable upon demand.

Interestingly, Stickgold (2005) notes that additional lines of investigation have provided converging evidence regarding the role of sleep in neural plasticity. Specifically, this involves observations of several genes that are upregulated during sleep, which are believed to contribute to neural plasticity and memory consolidation. Obviously, many more studies need to be carried out, with many more details to be inferred. However, the door to this mystery has finally been opened.

Parallel Distributed Processing and Emotion

The exploration of emotion forces us to confront two major problems. The first is the heterogeneity of phenomena that qualify to be included in this group. Although the argument continues, the majority of opinions appear to be that the range of emotional expression can be approximated by the following: happiness, lust, love, sadness, fear, anger, or disgust. No matter the individual particulars of the list, from a descriptive perspective, it can never be complete. The second problem, although not so complex, is the distinction between emotions and feelings.

Emotions Versus Feelings

Emotions are complicated, largely automated programs (neural maps) mediated by biological emotional action systems that have been constructed by and conserved through evolution. Recall that from its very evolutionary inception, mindedness (in this case, emotion) is the internalization of action. Therefore, the world of emotions is largely one of actions carried out in our bodies, from facial expressions and postures to changes in our viscera and internal physiological environment.

Feelings, on the other hand, are composite perceptions (or cognitive translations) of what is happening in our body while we are in the process of emoting, along with perceptions of our state of mind during that same period. Damasio (2010) argues that as far as the body is concerned, feelings are images of actions rather than the actions themselves. Accordingly, in simple organisms capable of behavior but not a mind process, emotions can be alive and well, but states of feeling may not necessarily follow. Regarding the interplay of emotions and feelings in humans, Damasio offers poetically,

> Emotions are the dutiful executors and servants of the value principle, the most intelligent offspring yet of biological value. On the other hand, emotion's own offspring, the emotional *feelings* that color our entire life from cradle to grave, loom large over humanity by making certain that *emotions are not ignored* [emphasis added]. (p. 108)

Emotional Operating Systems

Panksepp (1998) argues that the study of the brain in general and of emotions in particular must become rooted in the evolutionary realities of the brain if it is to be true science. Again, the theme of evolution's steady but subtle tinkering is invoked to underscore the foundational understanding that human functioning is only a variation of that found in lower animals. Accordingly, the emotional systems of the brain that create mixtures of innate and learned action tendencies in humans, as well as other creatures, must be studied in order to truly understand human affective (emotional) processes.

Emotions as FAPs

In parallel with this, Rodolfo Llinas (2001) proposes that we regard emotions as elements in the class of *fixed action patterns* (FAPs), where the actions are not motor but premotor. Furthermore, he recommends that we consider that, as with muscle tone, which serves as the basic platform for the execution of our movements, emotions represent the premotor platform that either drives or deters most of our actions. He argues,

> The relationship of emotional states to actions, and indeed to motricity, is all-important, for under normal conditions it is an emotional state that provides the trigger and internal context for action. But the underlying emotional state, the premotor FAP, does not only trigger the action as a FAP, it is also expressed in the form of another accompanying motor FAP, such as a facial expression, which telegraphs to others the context or motivation for the action and possibly the imminence of the action itself. (pp. 156–157)

Similarly, Damasio's (2010) dispositions contribute to emotional processes by generating actions of many kinds and many levels of complexity, such as the release of hormones into the bloodstream and the contraction of muscles in the viscera as well as muscles in the body, the face, or the vocal apparatus.

As an example, animals do not need to learn to search their environment for items needed for survival. A prewired program (neural map) for *seeking* is built into the brain. Also, animals do not need to learn to experience and express fear, anger, pain, lust, or joy. As we shall see, evolution has imprinted many *spontaneous neurobehavioral action patterns* within the inherited neural dynamics of the brains of most animals.

Consequently, Panksepp (1998) argues that "all mammals, indeed all organisms, come into the world with a variety of abilities that do not require previous learning, but which provide immediate opportunities for more complex learning to occur" (p. 25).

The Evolution of Biological Action Systems

With respect to emotion, Panksepp's (1998) emotional operating systems, Llinas's (2001) FAPs, and Damasio's (2010) dispositions offer solutions to such survival problems as the following: How do I obtain what I need? How do I safely keep what I need? How do I remain intact and safe? How do I make sure I have social contacts and supports? Such major survival questions, which all animals face, have been answered during the long course of neural evolution by the emergence of these intrinsic emotional neural tendencies (preset maps) within the brain.

Neural Criteria of Emotional Systems

Panksepp (1998) argues that from the perspective of affective neuroscience, it is essential to have neurally based definitions that can be utilized equally well in brain research and in the psychological and behavioral studies that are conducted on mature humans, infants, and other animals. Accordingly, Panksepp lists six objective neural criteria that define emotional operating systems, FAPs, and dispositions (action systems) in the brain. These criteria are as follows:

1. The underlying circuits must be genetically predetermined and designed to respond unconditionally to stimuli arising from major life-challenging circumstances.
2. These circuits must organize diverse behaviors by activating or inhibiting motor circuits and concurrent autonomic hormonal changes that have proved to be adaptive in the face of such life-challenging circumstances during the evolutionary history of the species.

3. These emotional circuits must change the sensitivities of sensory systems that are relevant to the behavioral sequences that have been aroused. In other words, they can modulate sensory inputs by making them more or less sensitive to incoming stimuli.
4. The neural activity of these emotional systems must outlast the precipitating circumstances, indicating their stability and consistency over time.
5. These emotional circuits must come under the conditional control of emotionally neutral environmental stimuli. In other words, they can be modulated by cognitive inputs, allowing the creature to acquire learned, conditioned responses to neutral environmental stimuli.
6. These circuits must have reciprocal interactions with the brain mechanisms that elaborate higher decision-making processes and consciousness.

These action systems are, therefore, self-organizing and self-stabilizing with respect to homeostasis, time, and context of experience. They are also functional systems that have been developed in the course of evolution and are analogous to mammalian and other species' biological systems.

Classifying Emotional Operating Systems

Panksepp (1998), utilizing descriptive rather than scientific names, designates the following emotional operating systems (action systems) as defined primarily by *genetically coded neural circuits* that generate well-organized emotional and behavioral sequences, which can be evoked by localized electrical stimulation of these neural circuits in the brain:

1. The seeking system, which mediates interest in and exploration of the environment, food seeking, warmth, and sexual gratification
2. The fear system, which mediates flight or freeze
3. The rage system, which mediates fight
4. The panic system, which mediates distress vocalization and social attachment

The Seeking System

This emotional system is a coherent neural network that mediates a certain category of survival abilities. This system makes animals *intensely interested* in exploring their world and leads them to become *excited* when they are about to get what they desire. It enables animals to find and eagerly anticipate the things they need for survival, such as food, water, warmth, and their ultimate evolutionary survival need, sex.

Ostensibly, when fully aroused, this system fills the mind with interest and motivates organisms to move their bodies effortlessly in search of the things they need, crave, and desire (Panksepp, 1998). In humans, this may likely be one of the main brain systems that generates and sustains *curiosity*, even for intellectual pursuits. In addition, this system is obviously efficient at facilitating learning, especially mastering information about where material resources are situated and the best way to obtain them.

The Rage System

Working in opposition to the seeking system is the system that mediates anger. Consequently, rage is aroused by frustration and attempts to curtail an animal's freedom of action. This system not only helps animals and humans to defend themselves but also energizes behavior when an animal or human is irritated or restrained.

The Fear System

Panksepp (1998) argues that the circuitry of this system was probably designed during evolution to help animals reduce pain and the possibility of destruction. Therefore, when stimulated, this circuit leads animals to run away. In addition, it provokes, in animals, a *freeze* response. This response can be sympathetic in nature, leading to a hyperaroused stillness (reducing the possibility of destruction), or parasympathetic in nature, leading to an immobility and analgesia (reducing the pain of an imminent destruction). In humans, this system operates in a similar manner, allowing us to be still or to escape into dissociative fugue states. More on this later.

The Panic System

As a result of this neural network, evolution has provided safeguards to assure that parents take care of their offspring, while giving their young and dependent offspring a powerful emotional system to indicate that they are in need of care (as reflected in crying and other separation calls).

These systems, therefore, are the basic elements that shape personality. Ideally, integration occurs within and among these action systems as a result of a nontraumatic developmental course. Over the course of evolution, these primitive action systems have become linked with higher cortical functions, enabling us to engage in complex action tendencies, including complex relationships (van der Hart, Nijenhuis, & Steele, 2006).

When the evolutionary growth of the human cortex opened up the relatively closed circuits of our mammalian and reptilian brains, we were enabled to consider alternatives of our own making rather than solely of nature's making. We could now choose to enjoy fear (if appropriate) or to create art out of our loneliness. Panksepp (1998) notes that "affectively, we can choose to be the angels or devils . . . we can choose to present ourselves in ways that are different from the ways we truly feel. We can be warm or acerbic, supportive or sarcastic, at will" (p. 301). However, it is unlikely that these sophisticated human feelings could exist without the basic neural scaffolding of our ancient emotional systems.

Functioning as adults therefore involves a profound complexity of biopsychosocial goals (caring for children, socializing, competing, loving, and protecting and exploring our inner and outer worlds). Meeting these goals involves a deep integration of these action systems. Indeed, most psychological conflicts, from the neurotic to the severely dissociative, involve the difficulty of balancing and integrating these action systems. We shall return to this.

Neural Circuitry of Emotional Operating Systems, FAPs, and Dispositions

The organizing system that integrates the emotional and biological realms of mind and body is the orbitofrontal cortex (OFC), located in the right hemisphere. This structure exerts executive management over the functioning of the entire right hemisphere. It sits at the apex of the rostral limbic system and mediates the functions of the anterior cingulate gyrus, thalamus, hypothalamus, insula, hippocampus, amygdala, mesencephalon, pons, and medulla oblongata.

Orbitofrontal Function and Structure

The OFC is known to play a crucial role in the processing of *interpersonal signals* required for the initiation of social interactions between individuals (Schore, 1994). Orbitofrontal neurons, in particular, process visual and auditory information associated with *emotionally* expressive faces and voices (Romanski et al., 1999; Scalaidhe, Wilson, & Goldman–Rakic, 1997). This frontolimbic system is also involved in the representation of highly integrated information on the organismic (body) state (Tucker, 1992). It is now thought that the most basic level of the regulatory process is the regulation of arousal (Tucker, Luu, & Pribram, 1995). Accordingly, the OFC, in the right hemisphere, is involved in both the generation and regulation of arousal (Critchley, Corfield, & Chandler, 2000). We will return to this in greater detail.

Ventral Sympathetic OFC

The ventral sympathetic frontal area of the OFC mediates dopaminergic arousal (Iversen, 1977). Recall that the dopaminergic system utilizes dopamine as its transmitter, binds to dopaminergic receptor sites, and mediates aspects of exploratory and seeking motor function, reward, cognition, and endocrine mechanisms.

This circuitry (the components of this neural map) begins in the reticular formations of the brainstem and projects rostrally (in a direction away from the brainstem, toward the cortex) to the sympathetic nuclei of the hypothalamus, to the amygdala, and then further up to the cingulate gyrus and, finally, the ventral frontal area of the OFC.

Recollect that the emotional operating systems (action systems) are defined primarily by specific, genetically coded neural circuits that generate well-organized emotional and behavioral sequences, which can be evoked by localized electrical stimulation of these neural circuits in the brain. Consequently, this excitatory (energy-expanding) limbic circuit, the *ventral tegmental limbic forebrain–midbrain circuit*, is involved with the generation of positively valenced states associated with approach behavior, motivational reward, and active coping strategies (Corbett & Wise, 1980; Schore, 1994, 2001a). Therefore, this circuitry contains the neural maps that mediate the seeking and panic systems, thereby, mediating our love affair with the world and the people around us. It also mediates the systems of rage and the sympathetically mediated flight aspects of the fear system, allowing us to actively fight or run away from danger.

Lateral Parasympathetic OFC

The lateral regions of the OFC have reciprocal connections with arousal-regulating noradrenergic neurons. This comprises the later-maturing (energy-conserving) limbic circuit, the *lateral tegmental limbic forebrain–midbrain circuit*, which activates the onset of a parasympathetic inhibitory state, regulates negative affect, and is associated with avoidance and passive coping (Nauta & Domesick, 1982; Schore, 1994, 2001a).

Stimulation of orbitofrontal noradrenergic inhibitory circuits results in "behavioral calming" (Arnsten, Steere, & Hunt, 1996). This circuitry (the components of this neural map) begins in the brainstem medulla (vagal complex), projecting rostrally to the parasympathetic nuclei of the hypothalamus and to the amygdala and the cingulate gyrus, finally ending in the lateral regions of the OFC. Accordingly, this circuitry contains the neural maps that mediate the parasympathetic aspects of the fear system, thereby enabling us to passively escape or cope with the events that frustrate our seeking and attachment, by mediating passive withdrawal or tonic immobility.

Orbitofrontal Cortex Excitation and Inhibition

In the orbitofrontal areas, *dopamine excites* and *norepinephrine inhibits* neuronal activity (mediating a calming effect). The functioning of these two limbic circuits in the OFC illustrates that emotions and the systems that mediate them organize behavior along a basic *appetitive–aversive* dimension associated with either a behavioral set involving *approach* (exploration, attachment, or aggression) or a set disposing *avoidance,* (passive escape and defense; Schore, 2001a). Therefore, these circuits mediate and organize the neural maps of the emotional operating systems, FAPs, and dispositions noted above. We will return to this in further detail.

Triggering and Executing Emotions

The fact that emotions are unlearned, automated, and predictably stable action programs illustrates their origin in natural selection and genetic instruction. Damasio (2010) opines that these instructions have been highly conserved by evolution and result in the brain being assembled in a particular, dependable way, such that certain neuronal circuits (neural maps) process emotionally based stimuli and facilitate the construction of full-fledged and adaptive emotional responses.

So, how are emotions triggered and executed? Generally, by images of objects or events that are actually happening in the moment or that have happened in the past and are now being recalled. Signals from the processed images are then made available to several regions of the brain, corresponding to the neural circuits noted above. Accordingly, certain configurations of signals (neural maps) are likely to activate one particular neural circuit while not activating others. As an example, depending on the context of the environmental (inner or outer) stimulus, neural maps become activated, making us feel happy, sad, angry, or fearful. On occasion, certain stimuli are vague enough to activate more than one site, facilitating a composite emotional state, resulting in a mixed feeling such as *bittersweetness.*

Emotional Triggering

In humans, emotions can trigger ideas and plans. As an example, a negative emotion such as sadness can lead to the recall of ideas about negative facts or memories, whereas a positive emotion can provoke the opposite. Accordingly, certain styles of mental processing are quickly instituted as an emotion develops. Sadness, for instance, slows down thinking and can provoke one to dwell on situations that incited it, whereas joy may accelerate thinking and reduce attention to unrelated events. The total of these responses constitutes an emotional state, unfolding rapidly and then subsiding until further stimuli capable of causing emotions are experienced. *Feelings* of emotions comprise the next step, constituting the composite perception of all that had gone on during the emotion.

Emotion programs utilize all the components of our life-regulatory machinery that have been conserved through evolution, such as the sensing and detection of conditions, the measurement of degrees of internal need, and our capacity for prediction. Damasio (2010) offers that "drives and motivation are simpler constituents of emotion. This is why one's happiness or sadness alters the state of one's drives and motivations, immediately changing one's mix of appetites and desires" (p. 111).

Emotional Execution

Recall that emotional memory and its resultant emotions are nondeclarative, in that emotional memory is derived from experience but is expressed as a change in behavior or emotional state rather than as a recollection. As we saw in the section on memory, many forms of nondeclarative memory are also well developed in invertebrate animals. These forms of learning, such as habituation, sensitization, and classical conditioning, have been preserved through evolutionary history and are present in all animals with a sufficiently developed nervous system, from invertebrates such as Aplysia (snails) and Drosophila (flies) to vertebrates, including humans (Squire & Kandel, 1999). Vertebrates have obviously evolved more complex forms of emotional and habitual learning, corresponding to their more complex perceptual emotional and motor repertoires.

These various forms of nondeclarative memory do not require the participation of the medial temporal lobe (hippocampal and parahippocampal) memory system. Consequently, we refer to nondeclarative memory and its resultant emotion as *reflexive* and to declarative memory and its resultant recollection as *reflective*. Squire and Kandel (1999) note,

> In no small part, by virtue of the unconscious status of these forms of memory, they create much of the mystery of human experience. Here arise the dispositions, habits, and preferences that are inaccessible to conscious recollection but that nevertheless are shaped by past events, influence our behavior and mental life, and are an important part of who we are. (p. 193)

Parallel Distributed Processing and Language

Rodolfo Llinas (2001) argues that language is the child of abstract thought. By itself, this statement does not sound very radical, given that many people consider abstraction and language as the exclusive sophisticated domains of humans. However, Llinas, grounded by scientific discipline, is well aware that, essentially, nothing in the functioning of human beings is purely unique to us from an evolutionary perspective. No matter how sophisticated any of our functions appear, they are only *upgrades*, the slight tinkering of evolution, and if we look carefully enough, we will find the origins and scaffolding of any particular human function in other vertebrates as well as invertebrates.

Abstraction

So, what do we mean by abstraction and/or abstract thinking? By and large, abstraction generally refers to something that exists only in the mind, an idea, a concept, a mental representation or image of something that may (or may not) exist in the outside world. Given what we have already seen with respect to evolution, abstraction or the group of neural processes that produce abstraction must be a fundamental principle of nervous system function.

In view of that, Llinas (2001) suggests that, as such, it is rather likely that abstract thinking probably began long ago in very primitive nervous systems. This view is supported by the observation that the nervous system is geared toward information processing, prediction, and action. Accordingly, in order for any animal to generate adaptive and predictive action, it must first be capable of generating some type of an internal image of itself, and this image must be the basis of a strategy around which to organize the tactics (prediction) of what the animal will do. Moreover, beyond the animal's sense of itself, physically, and the input that it receives from the external environment, the intrinsic circuits of its nervous system must be capable of generating an internal representation of its outside world in order for it to predict and act, by launching the appropriate FAPs. That sounds rather abstract, does it not?

Prosody: The Origin and Foundation of Language

So, what do we mean when we think of *language*? I would think that the first thing that comes to mind is human language, its variety, the fact that it is both spoken and written, and that it conveys abstraction and complexity. In addition, in the absence of an understanding of evolution, most people would consider it uniquely human. However, as we have already seen with respect to evolution's patterns, this cannot be. Although we do exhibit the richest and most complex of languages, we are neither the origin nor sole possessor of it.

Let us begin by defining language as a method by which one animal may communicate with another. Recall that Llinas (2001) has argued that language is a logical product of the intrinsic abstracting properties of the central nervous system. Accordingly, he posits that a foundational subcategory within language is *prosody*, a "form of motor behavior, an outward gesturing of an internal state, an outward expression of essentially generated abstraction that means something to another animal" (p. 229). For us, smiling, laughter, frowning, and the lifting of eyebrows are all FAPs and manners of prosody, for they communicate our internal, momentary state in a way that is familiar and understandable to others.

Prosody in Insects

Although not spoken, prosody is nonetheless language that is purposeful and communicative in its intent and function and by no means confined to humans. As an example, one of the first nonhuman languages to be understood was that of bees. Hammer and Menzel (1995) argue that this language is basically a dance, a rhythm and orientation performed in space. These varied dances, each specific to bees of a particular species, communicate information about the quantity and location of food, relative to the beehive. This constitutes a form of communication that requires a social order so that information conveyed may be utilized to some purpose by the receiving organism.

Prosody in Mammals

At a higher level of evolution, we can see languages that convey a more complex level of organization. In wolves, prosody is more sophisticated, utilizing numerous motor avenues for expression, including vocalization, eye contact, head gesturing, and whole-body communication. As an example, dominance is communicated both by the alpha male's expression of physical might as well as the subordinate males expressing their social position and submission by rolling over onto their back and offering the alpha male their neck. This form of language, mediated by premotor/emotional and motor FAPs, establishes a social hierarchy that is central to the strategies of the pack as a whole.

Human Language

Human language developed as an extension of these premotor conditions. As our abstract thinking grew richer, it became necessary for evolution to allow humans to override their existing FAPs, by adding increased circuitry and sophistication to their thalamocortical system. However, nature and evolution kept our basic FAPs as a foundation, while giving us the ability to elaborate on them. Thus, prosody is the foundation, and human language is the house we have built on it. Llinas (2001) suggests that "it is the finely achieved evolutionary balance between automatic computational efficiency and the ability to generate necessary nuance to our actions that characterizes the uniqueness of our brain and its abilities" (p. 242).

Let us examine, as an example, something like public speaking with respect to the number of neural systems that must be linked together in parallel [parallel distributed processing (PDP)]. Regarding neural motor systems, one must be able to maintain an erect vertical stance, at times pacing and moving, while executing systems that allow for respiratory, laryngeal, and orofacial mechanisms to act synchronously. Sensorial systems that mediate sensation and perception must come online. Simultaneously, associational, cognitive, memorial, and other neural systems that mediate thought and abstraction must be activated and linked. Finally, a neural system that interlaces FAPs with their sophisticated elaboration, mediating our elegant human language, must be activated. It is the total of this parallel and distributed processing and function that gives us human language.

Temporal Binding

As we have seen thus far, neural functions like perception, memory, language, and other aspects of consciousness are based on a highly distributed information processing system throughout the brain. One of the major questions, as yet, is how this information is synchronously integrated and how coherent representational states (temporal maps) can be established in the distributed neuronal systems (spatial maps) that subserve these functions.

In other words, PDP and connectionism inform us of the construction and mapped contents of these distributed neural systems. Parallel distributed processing mediates the activation of the required systems to be *linked* for any aspect of information processing (spatial mapping). How, then, do these systems, each created by the synchronization of action potentials, each oscillating at its own signature frequency, bind together to form coherent and integrated perceptual, memorial, somatosensory, linguistic, or emotional images and experiences (temporal maps)? Or, if PDP supplies the parts/systems to be linked, as well as the spatial map to their locations, what is it that facilitates the connection/binding of various systemic frequencies (into one common frequency), which is requisite for coherent and integrated (as opposed to fragmented) function and experience (temporal mapping)?

As we shall now see, it appears to be the thalamocortical circuitry and its inherent 40-Hz gamma-band activity that is required to bind, in real time, the various neuronal assemblies mentioned above, each oscillating at their own respective frequencies (Llinas, 2001; Llinas & Ribary, 2001; Singer, 1993, 2001).

Thalamocortical Temporal Binding of Specific and Nonspecific Thalamic Nuclei

In order to understand this complex and mysterious process, let us begin with an experiential example. Imagine, if you will, that you are at a scientific meeting, attending a talk. The next slide displayed shows a therapist and his patient who have both fallen asleep. You and the audience find yourselves laughing, but you know that there is more than humor being expressed. In an audience of psychotherapists, everyone is keenly aware that this was a complex experience, in that this laughter resonated both the humor of the moment and the fact that the scenario depicted in the slide is also considered to be a therapist's worst nightmare. Let us examine the role of temporal binding in this experience.

Temporal Binding of External Reality

A schematic of the thalamocortical circuitry that appears to subserve temporal binding is presented in Figure 5.1.

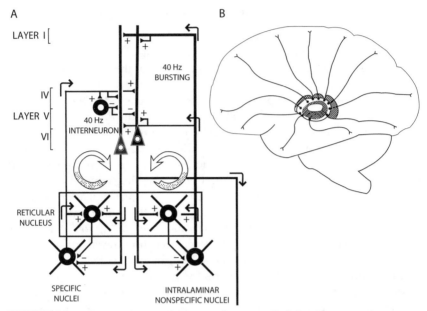

FIGURE 5.1   Diagram of two thalamocortical systems. (*Left*) Specific sensory or motor nuclei which mediate information from the external environment. (*Right*) Second loop shows nonspecific intralaminary nuclei which mediate information from our internal subjective environment.
Adapted from Llinas, R., & Ribary, U. (1993). Coherent 40 Hz oscillation characterizes dream state in humans. *Proceedings of the National Academy of Sciences, USA*, 90, 2078–2081. Copyright 1993, National Academy of Sciences, USA.

In response to your externally driven attention or perception (in this case, the slide), 40-Hz gamma-band oscillatory waves (in circuit A on the left side of Figure 5.1) generated by the "specific" ventrolateral and reticular thalamic nuclei would project to and establish resonance with the *sensorial* and *motoric* circuitry (each oscillating at its own signature frequencies) of neural layer IV. These 40-Hz oscillations would also establish resonance with other 40-Hz-wave-generating interneurons in layer IV. This 40-Hz oscillatory, wavelike activity would, in effect, *scan for, target, and synchronize* the frequency and activity of these sensory and motor systems (initially oscillating at their own signature frequencies), creating a *network frequency resonance*, thereby binding them into a coherent and integrated, externally generated perceptual experience.

Put another way, the complex spatial maps created by the functioning of your eyes, ears, nose, skin (tactile), and muscles, combined with their respective visual, auditory, olfactory, somatosensory, and motoric cortices, located in distant neural locations, would be synchronized into a coherent neural ensemble, simultaneously in real time, thereby synchronizing the neural systems that mediate your experience of information from the external world (temporal mapping).

These specific ventrolateral oscillations would then return and reenter the thalamus via layer VI, producing a *return feedback* in the *reticular* and *ventrolateral* thalamic nuclei (Llinas & Pare 1991; Llinas & Ribary, 2001; Singer, 1993; Steriade et al., 1990). In other words, the return of these oscillations to the thalamus would constitute the temporal map of the extrinsic (external) sensory information that was perceived with respect to the slide.

Temporal Binding of Internal Reality

Simultaneously, in circuit B (on the right side of Figure 5.1), 40-Hz gamma-band oscillatory waves, generated by the "nonspecific" central–lateral and reticular thalamic nuclei, would project to and establish resonance with the interoceptive neural circuits (spatial maps) mediating associations, memories, emotions, and other internal subjective phenomena (each oscillating at its own signature frequencies) of layers VI and I. These 40-Hz oscillations would also establish resonance with other 40-Hz-wave-generating interneurons in layers VI and I. This 40-Hz wavelike oscillatory activity would, in effect, scan for, target, and synchronize the activity of these inner interoceptive systems (initially oscillating at their own signature frequencies), creating a network frequency resonance, thereby binding them into a coherent and integrated, internally generated perceptual experience.

Put another way, the complex spatial maps created by the functioning of your associations, memories, and emotions, located in various neural locations, would be synchronized into a coherent neural ensemble (temporal map), simultaneously in real time, thereby synchronizing the neural systems that mediate your experience of information from your internal subjective world. Therefore, the areas of the brain that associated with and mediated the laughter, other emotions, memories, the meaning of patients and therapists falling asleep during sessions, and any other subjective experiences of the slide were connected to and bound together.

Temporal Binding of Combined Internal and External Realities

These nonspecific, central–lateral oscillations reenter the thalamus via layers V or VI to the reticular and central–lateral thalamic nuclei. The *simultaneous combined return* of gamma-band oscillations (from both circuits), into the thalamic reticular nuclei produces a *concurrent summation* (a combined temporal map) of the specific and nonspecific encoded and synchronized information, thereby enabling your integrated experience of the *extrinsic* sensory material, *intrinsic* laughter, and any other inner subjective experience that the slide produced.

The temporal binding studies noted above illustrate that the neural summation of these two overarching and global thalamocortical circuits produces the temporal binding that is required to generate coherent motor, perceptual, somatosensory, cognitive, emotional, memorial, and linguistic functioning. Therefore, the *specific* thalamocortical circuitry provides the *content* that relates to the external world, whereas the *nonspecific* thalamocortical circuitry provides the *context* (interoceptive subjective awareness) of any given moment of consciousness.

As in other areas of neural functioning, this model illustrates only the foundational contours of neural synchrony and binding. The exact details have yet to be inferred. How exactly does the brain's pervasive 40-Hz oscillatory activity modulate the frequency of parietal and temporal systems that tend to oscillate in the delta (0.1–3 Hz) and theta (3–8 Hz) ranges, of occipital systems that tend to oscillate in the alpha (8–12 Hz) range, or of parietal and frontal systems that tend to oscillate in the beta (12–30 Hz) range? How are these varying frequencies modulated, or in some way inhibited, in order to create a network frequency resonance that binds them coherently and temporally? If we note the lessons that evolution has taught us thus far, it is likely that the answer to these questions resides in some aspects of molecular genetics and protein synthesis. However, as in all things, first come the contours then eventually the details. Nonetheless, the contours are fascinating!

From Neurons to Self

Llinas (1987, 2001) has argued that the brain is predominantly a *closed* system, whose organization is geared primarily toward the generation of intrinsic (inner-generated) images. At first glance, that might not seem right. Should it not be an open system designed primarily to process information from the outside world, to deal with reality?

Until recently, in the absence of functional neuroimaging and its resultant data, the predominant view, as originally suggested by Sherrington (1906), had been that the brain was an open system, utilizing its energy to deal predominantly with outer reality. However, the recent research data have been refuting this notion. Yet, long before the newer data, William James (1890) presciently suggested the following:

> Enough has now been said to prove the general law of perception, which is this, that whilst part of what we perceive comes to our senses from the object before us, another part (and it may be the larger part) always comes (in Lazarus's phrase) out of our own head. (p. 103)

Although predominantly ignored by mainstream psychology, this notion did inspire Sigmund Freud and became the cornerstone of the psychoanalytic movement.

Neural Energy Consumption

So, what do the data illustrate? In the average adult human, the brain represents about 2% of the body weight. Remarkably, though, despite its relatively small size, the brain accounts for about 20% of the energy consumed by the entire body (Clark & Sokoloff, 1999; Raichle, 2006). Even more noteworthy, this high energy consumption occurs even in the *resting state*, a behavioral state characterized by quiet repose with eyes either closed or open and with or without visual stimulation. Furthermore, relative to this very high rate of energy consumption, the *additional* energy consumption associated with evoked changes in the brain (processing information from the external world) is remarkably small, often less than 5% (Raichle, 2006, 2009). Therefore, the overwhelming majority of the energy utilized by the brain is for our intrinsic inner reality, whereas only a small amount is utilized to deal with any aspect of our outer reality.

Marcus Raichle (2009), one of the pioneers of functional neuroimaging, notes that from these data, it appears clear that the brain's enormous energy consumption (mediated by intrinsic activity) is hardly affected by extrinsically mediated task performance. Noting his agreement with Llinas (2001), Raichle argues that evolution has designed and ordained that the majority of the brain's prediction is driven and mediated by its intrinsic and, therefore, *subjective* circuitry: not *objective* reality. It has long been suspected that the capability to reflect on the past or to ponder the future has facilitated the development of unique human attributes such as imagination and creativity. Indeed, there is nothing more human than the way that we utilize our subjective interpretation (intrinsic) of the past to generate predictions about our present and future.

Ostensibly, then, extrinsic information has much less value in our decisions about our personal life than it should. Recall that in order for the nervous system to predict, it must perform a rapid comparison of the sensory properties/input of the external world with a separate internal/subjective representation of the world. In humans, this internal representation is driven by sensorimotor experiences, associations, memories, and emotions. Therefore, this balance shifted toward inner subjectivity and the predictions that it generates about ourselves, our environment, and those around us, at the expense of outer objectivity, is at the heart of our knowledge, creativity, joys and sorrows, and the quality of our relationships.

Consequently, some have raised the intriguing possibility that the spontaneous, ongoing activity of the brain may actually generate, by design, globally coherent processes by itself. This brings us back to Rodolfo Llinas's (2001) notion that the brain is predominantly a closed system, whose organization is geared primarily toward the generation of intrinsic (inner-generated) images. Therefore, as a rule, sensory input from the external world (the specific side of the circuitry) is given its *significance* by the preexisting interoceptive *temperament* of the brain's internal subjective disposition (the nonspecific side of the circuitry).

Therefore, by design, our circuitry places a markedly higher priority on subjectivity than on objectivity. As clinicians, we certainly know that to be true. The majority of emotional problems that befall us, from neuroses to personality disorders to posttraumatic and dissociative disorders, are driven by intrinsic emotional perceptions that are no longer accurately congruent with extrinsic reality. It certainly begs the question as to whether our consciousness, intrinsic as it is by design, is adaptive or, indeed, an evolutionary *flaw* yet to be tinkered with. We will return to this.

The Essence of Consciousness

Recall that intrinsic subjectivity is mediated by the nonspecific circuitry of the thalamocortical system. Damage to nuclei of the specific thalamocortical system produces only a loss of the particular sensory modality that was mediated by the specific damaged nucleus. However, following damage to nuclei of the nonspecific thalamocortical system, all perception and, therefore, consciousness ceases. All extrinsic information mediated by the specific circuitry of the system can no longer be perceived or responded to (Llinas & Ribary, 2001; Llinas, 2001). Llinas opines,

> In essence, the individual no longer exists, from a cognitive point of view, and although specific sensory inputs to the cortex remain intact, they are completely ignored. These results argue that the nonspecific system is required to achieve binding, that is, to place the representation of specific sensory images into the context of ongoing activities. (p. 127)

Forty-Hertz Activity and Sleep

Recall that REM and non-REM sleep serve related but distinct functions in off-line memory processing, with non-REM sleep appearing most critical for strengthening of hippocampal episodic memories and REM sleep for the creation and strengthening of neocortical semantic memories. Therefore, if cognition is essentially an intrinsically generated state, what, if any, distinction is there between sleep and wakefulness? If cognition is a function of the 40-Hz thalamocortical resonance discussed above, what do we see regarding this oscillatory rhythm during sleep?

In a series of studies, Rodolfo Llinas and colleagues (Llinas & Pare, 1991; Llinas & Ribary, 1993), utilizing magnetoencephalography, studied 40-Hz resonance during wakefulness and sleep. They found that 40-Hz coherent activity was spontaneously present in the awake and REM sleep state. Interestingly, this 40-Hz resonance was markedly reduced during delta sleep. Of equal interest, an auditory stimulus produced well-defined 40-Hz oscillation in the wakeful state but none in either the delta or REM sleep states.

Llinas (2001) argues that two salient findings from these studies stand out. One is that the waking and REM sleep states are electrically very similar with respect to the presence of 40-Hz oscillations. The second is that 40-Hz oscillations are not reset by sensory input (i.e., an auditory signal) during REM sleep. Therefore, we do not perceive the external world during REM sleep, because the intrinsic activity of the nervous system is, evidently, considered paramount.

So, what exactly does this signify? Truthfully, we do not, as yet, know. Nonetheless, what is clear is that off-line information processing, manifested by delta (non-REM) and REM sleep states, requires an apparently exclusive intrinsic neural environment. Hence, evolution's preference for intrinsic elements of consciousness and its inherent information processing is again evident.

Self-Emergence

Reflection on the foregoing illustrates that the thalamocortical circuitry works as a closed system: a neural scaffolding that synchronously relates the sensory-referred properties of the external world to internally generated associations, emotions, motivations, and memories. Llinas (2001) argues that "this temporally coherent event that binds, in the time domain, the fractured components of external and internal reality to a single construct is what we call the *self*" (p. 126). Therefore, the self, Llinas's "I of the vortex," appears to us as an organizer of extrinsically and intrinsically derived images: the loom that weaves together that which is within and without us.

René Descartes (1644), in attempting to describe the self, wrote, "*Dubito, ergo cogito* [I doubt, therefore I think]; *cogito, ergo sum* [I think, therefore I am]." Rodolfo Llinas (2001) offers an update—It binds, therefore I am!

CHAPTER 6

Human Development

The forgoing examination of the neural substrates of information processing will serve as a platform from which we will examine the expression of numerous disruptions of consciousness.

In addition, given that a number of disorders of consciousness are developmental in origin, that is, they are occurring during human neural maturation and growth, another platform—that of human development must first be illustrated in order for us to fully realize the myriad spectrum of the disrepair of consciousness.

THE RIGHT HEMISPHERE

Allan Schore (1994, 2001a, 2001b, 2003a) maintains that the inceptive stages of development represent specifically a maturational period of the early-maturing right brain, which is dominant in the first 3 years of human life. The right brain is centrally involved not only in processing social–emotional information, promoting attachment functions, and regulating bodily and affective states, but also in the organization of vital functions supporting survival and enabling the organism to cope dynamically with stress (Whittling & Schweiger, 1993). The maturation of these adaptive right-brain regulatory capacities is *experience dependent*, embedded in the attachment connection between the infant and primary caregiver.

Thus, attachment theory is in essence an *affect-regulatory* theory (Schore, 1994, 2001a, 2001b). More specifically, in attachment transactions, the secure mother, at an intuitive unconscious level, is continuously regulating the baby's labile arousal levels and, therefore, emotional states. Ostensibly, the mother appears to provide an unconsciously mediated *neural synchronization* of her right hemisphere with the underdeveloped right hemisphere of her child.

Visual Stimulation, Neural Synchrony, and Neural Development

So, you might ask, how do mother and child synchronize their right hemispheres? As we have seen thus far, there is widespread evidence that the brain is an intrinsic, self-organizing system. However, there is perhaps less of an appreciation of the fact that the self-organization of the developing brain *must* occur in the context of a relationship with another brain (Schore, 2003a). Further, as we have already observed with respect to information processing, it must be undertaken in the context of *action*, not *passivity* (i.e., in sensorimotor form).

Visual Gaze

From the moment of birth, the child uses its maturing sensory capacities, especially taste, smell, and touch, to interact with the social environment. By the end of the second month, with the development and myelination (the electrically insulating material that forms a layer, the myelin sheath, around the axon of a neuron) of occipital areas involved in the visual perception of the human face, a dramatic progression of its social and emotional capacities becomes evident.

Mother and child begin the *symbiotic phase* of the separation–individuation process (Mahler, 1967). It is interesting that Margaret Mahler, a pioneer of developmental psychoanalytic research, in the absence of available neurobiological data, referred to the symbiosis of mother and child as a metaphor. As we shall soon realize, this appears not to be the case. Hence, over the first year of life, *visual* experiences play a major role in social and emotional development (Schore, 1994). The mother's emotionally expressive face is by far the most potent visual stimulus in the infant's environment, and the child's intense interest in her face, especially in her *eyes*, leads him to track it in space and to engage in periods of intense *mutual gaze*. In sustained joint gaze transactions,

> The mother's facial expression stimulates and amplifies positive affect in the infant. The child's internally pleasurable state is communicated back to the mother, and in this *interactive system of reciprocal stimulation* [emphasis added], both members of the dyad enter into a *symbiotic* [emphasis added] state of heightened positive affect. (p. 71)

The First Psychic Organizer

Research on face scanning indicates that infants are most sensitive to facial affective expressions in which specifically, the eyes have the most impact (Haith, Bergman, & Moore, 1979). By the age of 17 weeks, the eyes are a more salient feature of the mother's face than her mouth. By 2 to 3 months of age, the infant's smile can be induced by a full-faced presentation or a pair of circles painted on a balloon simulating the gestalt of a face. This smile can be quickly extinguished by the turning of the head so as to present the profile in which the representations of the eyes are eliminated. Rene Spitz (1965) notes,

Beginning with the second month of life, the human face becomes a privileged percept, preferred to all other things of the infant environment. Now, the infant is able to segregate and distinguish it from the background .... in the third month, this 'turning outward' in response to the stimulus of the human face, culminates in the new clearly defined, *species-specific* [emphasis added] response ... he will now respond to the adult's face with a smile. (p. 86)

Spitz referred to this *smile* as the first psychic *organizer* of the personality. Borrowing from embryology, wherein certain anatomical parts of embryos (referred to as organizers) must be present to induce the formation of other more advanced tissues or structures, Spitz believed that certain maturational and developmental milestones in the infant's development acted in the same epigenetic manner. Each was required to pave the way for the next.

Schore (1994), citing the work of Hess (1975), argues that the nature of pupil size in nonverbal communication may reveal the specific dynamics of mutual gaze and may elucidate the mechanisms by which the social environment operates to generate and amplify infant affect. In a series of studies, Hess found that one person uses another's pupil size as a source of information about that person's feelings or attitudes and that this process occurs at an unconscious level.

These experiments also illustrated that women's eyes dilate in response to a picture of a baby. Most important, Hess (1975) discovered that viewing enlarged dilated pupils rapidly elicited larger dilated pupils in the observer. Further, infants smiled more when the experimenter's eyes were dilated (a positively valenced sympathetic response) rather than constricted (a negatively valenced parasympathetic response), suggesting that dilated pupils act as a *releaser* in infants, triggering a response that is learned early in life. He also observed that dilated pupils in the infant *release* caregiver behavior. Accordingly, Schore (1994) argues that "the child thus fixates directly on the *visible portion of the mother's central nervous system* [emphasis added], her eyes, which specifically reflect the activity and state of her right hemisphere, the hemisphere that is known to be dominant for gaze behavior" (p. 75). He opines further, "I propose that during these eye to eye transactions the infant's maturing right hemisphere is psycho-biologically attuned to the output of the mother's right hemisphere" (p. 76).

Attachment and Affect Regulation

Damasio (1998) maintains that emotion and the experience of emotion are the highest-order direct expressions of bioregulation in complex organisms. Put another way, emotion is the most basic and yet complex expression of affective homeostatic regulation. Consequently, attachment and its inherent synchronization of maternal and infant right hemispheres are geared *fundamentally* toward affective regulation.

Accordingly, Schore (2001a) argues that dyadic affect regulation does not just consist of the reduction of affective intensity, such as the dampening of negative emotion, but also, and more important, involves the *amplification and intensification* of positively valenced (charged) emotion, the condition *most* necessary for complex developmental self-organization. Hence, attachment is not just the establishment of security after a dysregulating experience and stressful negative state but also, more important, an interactive amplification of positive affects resulting from gazing and plays states. Schore notes further,

> Regulated affective interactions with a familiar, predictable primary caregiver create not only a sense of safety, but also a *positively charged curiosity* [emphasis added] that fuels the burgeoning self's exploration of novel socio-emotional and physical environments. This ability constitutes a *marker* [emphasis added] of adaptive infant mental health. (p. 21)

Emotional Action Systems

If we recall the primacy of the emotional action systems (Panksepp, 1998), particularly seeking and panic, and their inherent *positively* valenced affective and *appetitive* nature, the importance of positive affects with respect to neural development becomes clearer.

Recollect that the seeking system mediates and motivates us to search for the things we need, crave, and desire. In addition, it may likely be one of the main brain systems that generates and sustains curiosity. As a consequence, it facilitates learning, especially mastering information about where material resources are situated and the best way to obtain them.

In the panic system, evolution has provided safeguards to assure that parents take care of their offspring, while giving their young and dependent offspring a powerful emotional system to indicate that they are in need of care (as reflected in *paniclike* crying and other separation calls). As we move beyond infancy into toddlerhood, it mediates our various levels of attachments as we progress into latency, adolescence, and adulthood.

So, how does sustained positive affect contribute to the development and organization of the seeking and panic systems? Another way of asking this question is as follows: What psychoneurobiological mechanism could underlie this caregiver-induced neural development and organization of the infant brain? The infant's response of positively valenced excitation, in response to the mother's face and other aspects of her own positively valenced excitation, generates high levels of dopaminergic-driven arousal and elation in the infant's right brain (Besson & Louilot, 1995).

Dopaminergic Arousal

Recall that the dopaminergic system utilizes dopamine as its transmitter, binds to dopaminergic receptor sites, and mediates aspects of motor function, positively valenced (charged) arousal, exploration, reward, cognition, and endocrine mechanisms. In addition, as we noted above, the ventral sympathetic frontal area of the orbitofrontal cortex (described in Chapter 5) mediates dopaminergic arousal and is centrally involved in motivated behavior, exploration, the nonverbal decoding of positive facial expressions, and mechanisms of pleasurable reward and motivation.

Consequently, this excitatory orbitofrontal circuit is involved with the generation of positively valenced states associated with approach behavior, motivational reward, and active coping strategies. Accordingly, this circuitry contains the neural maps that mediate the appetitive seeking and panic systems, thereby mediating our love affair with the world and the people around us. Schore (2001a) maintains that the bursting (machine-gun-like firing) of these dopaminergic neurons, in response to salient, positively arousing environmental stimuli, contributes to an orienting response, the setting of a heightened motivational state, and the onset of appetitive curiosity and exploratory behavior. We will return to orienting responses in detail.

Attachment, Play, and Neural Growth

Schore (2001a) maintains that the right hemisphere is also dominant for the perception of *biological motion* and that these psychoneurobiological actions of mother–infant play sequences drive the affective bursts embedded within moments of affective synchrony (of caretaker and infant's right hemispheres), in which positive states of *attention* and *delight* are dyadically amplified. Panksepp (1998) contends that "play may have direct *trophic* effects on neuronal and synaptic growth in many brain systems" (p. 296) and suggests that play serves the adaptive role of organizing affective information in emotional circuits. Trophism, in this case, refers to neural growth promotion, wherein *trophy* is the opposite of *atrophy*.

Play and Neural Growth

So, how can early play episodes account for and contribute to trophic neural effects? Schore (1994) argues that in these face-to-face emotional communications, the visual input of the mother's face and eyes is also inducing the production of *neurotrophins*, a family of proteins that induce the survival, development, and growth of neurons. Also known as *neurotrophic factors*, they belong to a class of growth factor proteins that are capable of signaling particular cells to survive, differentiate, or grow.

Brain-derived neurotrophic factor (BDNF), found mostly in the brain but also in the peripheral nervous system, acts to support the survival of existing neurons and promotes the growth and differentiation of new neurons and synapses. BDNF has been shown to be one of the most active neurotrophins involved in synaptogenesis (the creation of new synaptic connections).

Maternal care has been shown to increase amino acid (N-methyl-D-aspartate) receptor levels, resulting in elevated BDNF levels and synaptogenesis in the infant's brain (Liu, Diorio, Day, Francis, & Meany, 2000). In other words, this neural growth-promoting amino acid, which is stimulated and maintained by visual input and its resultant positive-affect enhancement (Gomez–Pinilla, Choi, & Ryba, 1999), is essential in the promotion of synaptic plasticity and growth during these critical periods of neural maturation and development (Huang et al., 1999). Again, we witness the critical relationship between interactive, positively valenced attachment and neural growth.

Attachment, Play, and Endorphins

Schore (1994) points out that, ironically, despite the existing knowledge regarding the intrinsic dyadic nature of the attachment-mediated synchronization of mother and child's right hemispheres, hardly any research has *concurrently* measured mother and infant in the process of interacting with each other. In one of the few studies of this kind, the data indicate that the intimate contact between the mother and her infant is mutually regulated by the reciprocal activation of their opiate systems, as elevated levels of beta-endorphins increase pleasure in both brains, simultaneously (Kalin, Shelton, & Lynn, 1995). Indeed, research has established that opioids enhance play behavior and that endorphins increase the firing of dopaminergic neurons (Yoshida et al., 1993). Hence, a cyclical pattern of pleasurable play and endorphin and dopamine release ensues.

Attachment and Practicing—Transitions Within Symbiosis

A dramatic biobehavioral shift occurs at the end of the first year of infancy, expressed in the cognitive, motor, and affective domains. The onset of the *practicing period* is defined by Mahler (1972) as consisting of rapid developmental changes in motor behavior, manifested by upright posture and locomotion, supporting the child's first and independent steps, an event *paramount* in human individuation. Schore (1994) opines that despite the significant motor, cognitive, and behavioral advances, it is the *affective* characteristics of this period that are unique and definitional.

Mahler (1972) describes the practicing period as consisting of two parts: (a) the early practicing phase, characterized by the infant's earliest ability to move away physically from the mother by crawling, climbing, and righting himself, while still holding on; and (b) the practicing period proper, characterized by free upright locomotion. Hence, this change is not only maturational (driven by new neurophysiological abilities) but also developmental (driven by neuropsychological progress and needs), in that it heralds the psychological hatching of the baby as she begins to move tentatively away from the symbiotic orbit with her mother.

Mahler (1972) notes,

> With the child's spurt in autonomous functions, especially upright locomotion, the 'love affair with world' is at its height. During these precious six to eight months (from ten–twelve to sixteen–eighteen months), for the junior toddler the world is his oyster . . . . the child seems intoxicated with his own faculties and with the greatness of his world. (p. 126)

During this time, the child appears impervious to knocks and falls. Driven by the maturation of his locomotor apparatus, the child ventures farther and farther away from the mother's feet, often so absorbed by his own activities that for long periods of time, he appears to be oblivious to her presence or absence. However, the child returns periodically to the mother, seeming to need her physical proximity and *refueling* from time to time.

Ontogenesis and Adaptation

Ontogenesis refers to the sequence of events involved in the development of an individual organism from its conception to its death. This maturational and developmental history involves the movement from simplicity to higher complexity. Ontogenesis is distinguished from phylogenesis, which refers to the evolutionary history of a genetically related group of organisms. According to the developmental biological concept of ontogenetic adaptation, developing capacities are specifically adaptive to the period in which they first emerge. In other words, certain developmental changes that may appear to be regressive (i.e., increased separation anxiety) will actually be adaptive, given the nature of the child's development at that specific time. We return to this in further detail below.

Accordingly, Schore (1994) argues that the affective, behavioral, and cognitive aspects that are unique to this period "reflect a biologically timed period of sympathetic-dominant limbic hyperarousal and behavioral over-excitation which have adaptive significance" (p. 95). He maintains further that developmental observers have noted that by 1 year of age, *stimulus-seeking exploratory* playtime increases to as much as 6 hours of the child's day. Ontogenetically, this change has numerous implications. Recall that heightened states of positively valenced (charged) affect and delight, which are sympathetic and dopamine driven, have been shown to increase amino acid (N-methyl-D-aspartate) receptor levels, resulting in elevated levels of brain-derived neurotrophic factor, both required for synaptogenesis (neural growth and wiring) in the infant's brain (Liu et al., 2000). In addition, this change heralds the first active manifestation of the seeking system, thereby setting a neuroemotional tone or template as the infant begins to *actively* explore his world.

The Second Organizer

Finally, this developmental period heralds the second organizer of the personality. Recall that certain maturational and developmental milestones in the infant are required to pave the way for the next more advanced milestone. Given that they are evident in all infants and toddlers, they are regarded as universal organizers of the self. Consequently, their presence signifies appropriate development, whereas their absence indicates lags or distortions in development.

Eight-Month Anxiety

With the advent of this organizer, *8-month anxiety*, the infant no longer responds with a smile when just *any* smiling visitor steps up to crib (Spitz, 1965). The child is now clearly able to distinguish friend from stranger. If a stranger does approach, it releases an unmistakable, characteristic behavior in the child, manifested by varying intensities of apprehension, anxiety, and rejection of the stranger. Recall that this is in contrast to the 3-month-old, for whom one human face is as good as another and for whom a balloon with eyes drawn on it produces the same *smile* (the first organizer) as her mother's face. Now, the stranger's face is compared to the memory of the mother's or other caretakers' faces, found to be different, and rejected. Hence, at this age, the baby is now able to recognize the caretaking *object* and shows evidence of increased imprinting and attachment.

Throughout this time, the child's regulated affective interactions with the familiar, predictable primary caregiver continue to create not only a sense of safety but also the positively charged *curiosity* that fuels the burgeoning self's exploration of novel socioemotional and physical environments. This ability continues to be a marker of adaptive infant mental health. In addition, this is taking place at a time when the child's sympathetic nervous system (SNS) is becoming increasingly active, whereas the parasympathetic (neurally inhibiting) part of the orbitofrontal cortex has yet to develop. Hence, the mother must continue to function as the child's inhibitory cortex. Schore (1994) opines,

> The practicing phase in which the infant truly becomes a behaviorally and socially dynamic organism represents a critical period for the formation of enduring attachment bonds to the primary caregivers. The nature of the attachment to the mother influences all later socio-emotional transactions. (p. 98)

Internal Imaging

At the end of the child's first year, the socioaffective transactions with the primary caregiver facilitate the growth, development, and stabilization of the neural interconnections between the memory-mediating anterior temporal lobe areas and the orbitofrontal cortex. Schore (1994) argues,

With this linkage, a visuo-limbic pathway is established . . . as a result, the infant creates a schema of the face of the attachment object . . . . this internal affect-associated image (internalized object relation) can be accessed even in the mother's absence, and is therefore an important mechanism of attachment functioning. (p. 175)

Consequently, the child's prefrontal system can now generate *interactive representations*, which function as nonverbal internal working models of the infant's transactions with the primary attachment figure that can now be accessed for *limited* regulatory purposes, even in the caretaker's absence. Hence, this emergent online connection between the infant's temporal memory and emotion-mediating centers and the visuoaffective centers of the orbitofrontal cortex enable the development of object permanence, allowing the infant to now be able to *carry his caretakers around in his mind.*

Affect Regulation in the Second Year

In optimal growth-promoting environments, the interactive mechanism for generating positive affect becomes profoundly efficient, allowing the toddler to experience very high levels of elation and excitement. Developmental studies reveal a marked increase in positive emotions from 10 to 13.5 months of age. As the practicing stage comes to an end, the socioemotional environment of the caregiver–infant dyad will change dramatically.

Parental Socialization

At 10 months of age, 90% of maternal behavior consists of affection, playing, and caregiving. In sharp contrast, however, the mother of the 13- to 17-month-old toddler now expresses a prohibition on an average of every 9 minutes (Rothbart, Taylor, & Tucker, 1989). Ostensibly, then, in the second year, the caretaker's role changes from solely a caregiver to a *socializing agent*, as she must now begin to persuade her child to inhibit unrestricted exploration, tantrums, and bladder and bowel functions, all activities that he enjoys (Schore, 2003a).

During this period, resulting from a rapid increase in cognitive and neuromuscular development, the child begins frequently to get into things and behave in ways that are at variance with parental desires. Consequently, his relationship with his caregivers begins to change, as they now attempt at socializing him by changing his behavior against his will, whereas he attempts to have his way. Thus, the stage is now set for sustained conflicts of will, thereby changing parental roles dramatically from primarily caretaking to increasingly socializing. For the child, the previously learned excited expectation of psychobiological attuned positive affect is now, at times, replaced with parental limit setting, resulting in confusion, anger, and shame.

Schore (2003a) notes that "in such a psychobiological state transition, sympathetically powered elation, high arousal, and elevated activity levels instantly evaporate. This represents a shift into a low-keyed inhibitory state of parasympathetic conservation and withdrawal" (p. 18). Hence, constant euphoria now gives way to unexpected disappointment and confusion. This state change is mediated by a different psychobiological pattern, wherein corticosteroids are now produced as a stress response. This change, then, reduces the endorphins and dopaminergic aspects of the positive-affect state. Therefore, as opposed to the previous constant positive-affect state, shame now elicits a painful infant distress state, manifested in a sudden decrement in pleasure, a rapid inhibition of excitement, and cardiac deceleration, due to an immature vagal complex in the medulla. Put another way, the previous constant elation and euphoria is now interrupted by disappointment and shame, ostensibly blowing the air out of the bubble of joy and omnipotence.

Parasympathetic Development

With respect to the child's maturation and development, this shift reflects the reduced activation of the sympathetic, excitatory circuitry and the increased activation and development of the parasympathetic, inhibitory circuitry. We will return to this and vagal function in detail below.

As a result of these new environmental and parental demands, the toddler is suddenly and unexpectedly propelled from the previously ongoing symbiotic positive-affective state into a negative affective state, a stressful state transition that he cannot autoregulate. Prolonged states of shame are too toxic for the infant to sustain for long periods of time. Hence, parental active participation in regulating and soothing the child's affect is critical to enabling the child to shift from the negative affective state of deflation and distress to a reestablished state of positive affect. In these early developmental periods, as the infant's affect-regulatory centers and capacities are developing, parents *must* provide for and facilitate the necessary modulation and regulation of emotional states, especially after disruptions of positive-affect states and during more subtle transitions. It is this continued parental regulation of the child's emotional state that eventually allows for the development of self-regulation.

If the caregiver is "sensitive, responsive, and emotionally approachable, especially if she reinstates and reenters into synchronized mutual-gaze visual-affect regulating transactions, the dyad is psychobiologically reattuned, shame is metabolized and regulated, and the attachment bond is reconnected" (Schore, 2003a, p. 19). This essential pattern of affect-regulatory *disruption and repair* (already foretelling the normal vicissitudes of life) creates interventions by the parents that allow for state transitions in the child. Hence, "the parasympathetic-dominant arousal of the shame state is supplanted by the re-ignition of sympathetic-dominant arousal that supports increased activity and positive affect" (Schore, p. 10). Consequently, this resumes corticotrophin release factor (CRF) and endorphin production and reactivates the excitatory circuitry. In this manner, the parent and infant dyadically negotiate stressful state transitions of emotion, cognition, and behavior. This creates an implicit-memory template for the endurance and conquering of negative experience, a template for interactive repair in the context of attachment.

The Third Organizer

In the midst of all the disruption and repair, the child's development contin-ues with respect to his transition from a symbiotic state to one of separation and individuation. As his unconscious awareness of separateness develops, the third organizer (Spitz, 1965), the *shaking of the head* and the utterance of "no," makes its appearance, heralding the onset of the "terrible twos." Spitz refers to this as the first "semantic gesture," the first adultlike communication. Many interpretations have been offered regarding the true nature of this ges-ture, ranging from imitation to identification with the aggressor. Blanck and Blanck (1974) argue elegantly that with this gesture, *action* is replaced by a semantic message that enhances the child's distinction between *self* and *object*. In either case, what appears most salient, though, is that saying "no" and refusing to comply with one's caretakers is the first expression of a *difference of opinion*, a child's way of expressing clearly, in the absence of adult language, that disagreement implies the emergent presence of a self that disagrees with the object. Hence, two opinions preclude the possibility of symbiotic merger, in that it takes two to disagree.

Rapprochement

This new awareness and insistence of separateness, combined with increased cognitive capacities, begins the provocation of a simultaneous separation–anxiety in the child. His previous relative obliviousness of his caretakers fades. His newfound separateness and his emerging nonconscious understanding of its implication is no longer just exhilarating but now also anxiety provok-ing. The earlier brief refueling contacts with his caretaker are now replaced with an increased need to interact and maintain contact, a phenomenon that Margaret Mahler (1972) referred to as *rapprochement*, the insistent need for increased reunion by the infant.

It is in this maturational milestone that we first observe developmental changes that may appear to be regressive (i.e., increased separation anxiety) but are actually adaptive, given the nature of the child's development at this specific time. Hence, the perception of one's separateness (a developmental growth) provokes, for the moment, an increase in anxiety and an *apparent* decrease in autonomy. Yet, this temporary manifestation of a seeming regression is adaptive and extremely necessary for the child's psychological growth, in that it signifies an increase in cognitive awareness that is, simultaneously, frightening.

As we noted, throughout these developmental shifts, parental active participation in regulating and soothing the child's affect is critical in enabling the child to shift from the negative affective state of distress to a reestablished state of positive affect. Recall that the self-organization of the developing brain must occur in the context of a relationship with another brain, in order to mediate what the child's brain cannot, as yet, execute.

Maturation and Development of Neural Inhibition

Schore (1994) argues that the stress of parental socialization and its inherent change in brain chemistry appear to define and provoke the optimal socioemotional stimulation required for further structural growth of the child's orbitofrontal cortex. Consequently, as a result of the inherent alternating disruption and repair of the attachment bond, the increase in noradrenergic (noradrenalin) input, combined with the decrease in endorphins, begins to mediate a reduction in the growth of the sympathetic dopaminergic system, heralding the increase in development and growth of the parasympathetic noradrenergic system.

In the same manner that the catecholamine dopamine was crucial in mediating the neurotrophism (neural growth and development) of the sympathetic circuitry, the catecholamine noradrenalin is now, vital in the neurotrophic growth of the parasympathetic circuitry (Felten, Hallman, & Jonsson, 1982; Schore, 1994). Consequently, the growth and expansion of axons from noradrenergic sites in the orbitofrontal cortex to subcortical targets in the medulla allow for noradrenaline's role in *vagal restraint* and the subsequent energy-conserving inhibition of sympathetic autonomic function.

To put it another way, the child's caregivers responding to his first developmental need for limit setting produce in the child frustration and shame and a resultant neurochemical change in predominant neurotransmission. Whereas the previous dominance of dopamine was crucial to the growth of the sympathetic (excitatory) circuitry, the current increasing presence of norepineprine/noradrenalin, provoked by the frustration and shame, is now essential for the growth of the parasympathetic, neural-inhibitory, and affect-regulatory circuitry. Again, we witness the profound effect of the attachment interaction on neural development, as well as the precise and timely attunement that is required in the caregivers, in order for this neurointeractive vortex to ensue adaptively.

So, how would the growth and expansion of this area of the orbitofrontal cortex into the brainstem medulla facilitate neural inhibition and emotional regulation? As we have seen thus far, emotional regulation and attachment seem to go hand in hand. Hence, attachment theory is essentially an affect-regulatory theory, with the self-organization of the developing brain occurring only in the context of a relationship with *another* brain.

The Vagus Nerve and Polyvagal Function

Stephen Porges (1997, 2001) maintains that in order to survive, mammals must communicate with their caretaking and social unit, determine friend from foe, and evaluate whether their environment is safe or not. With respect to development and beyond, "these survival related behaviors are associated with specific neurobiological states that limit the extent to which a mammal can be physically approached and whether the mammal can communicate or establish new coalitions" (2001, p. 124). In most mammals, but especially humans, this is predicated by affective (emotional) regulation. We return to this below.

Porges (1997, 2001) illustrates that embedded in the mammalian nervous system, are neuroanatomical structures related to the expression and experience of social and emotional behavior. As evolutionary forces molded the human nervous system, these new structures were added, and older structures were modified to allow greater dynamic range and finer control of physiological states and to facilitate the emergence of new, adaptive face-to-face social function, thereby distinguishing mammals and humans from reptiles and other vertebrates (Porges, 2011).

Vagal Evolution and Development

Several of these structures are shared with other vertebrates and represent the product of phylogenic (evolutionary course of a species) development. Via evolutionary processes, the mammalian nervous system has emerged with specific features that react to environmental challenge (situational or attachment driven) in order to maintain homeostasis. These reactions alter physiological state and, in mammals, mediate sensory awareness, motor behaviors, and cognitive potentials. In other words, these features allow for the increased sophistication and complexity of mammalian and human social interactions and attachment.

This evolution of the autonomic nervous system provides substrates (underlying mechanisms) for the emergence of three adaptive stress-coping subsystems, each coupled with structures that evolved during identifiable phylogenic stages. Porges (1997, 2001) refers to these systems as "polyvagal" to highlight and detail the neurophysiological and neuroanatomical distinction between two branches of the 10th cranial nerve (the vagus) and to propose that each vagal branch is associated with a different adaptive behavioral strategy.

The Vagus Nerve

The vagus nerve, a primary component of the autonomic nervous system, located in the brainstem medulla, is composed of branches that regulate the striated muscles of the head and face (facial muscles, eyelids, middle-ear muscles, larynx, pharynx, muscles of mastication) and in several visceral organs, such as the heart, lungs, and gut. The three branches of the polyvagal system, in ascending order of phylogenic development (from most primitive to advanced), are as follows:

1. The *dorsal vagal complex* is situated in the dorsal motor nucleus of the medulla, a parasympathetic system that is a vestigial *immobilization* mechanism. In humans, through rapid lowering of cardiac and respiratory function, it mediates the shutdown of metabolic activity, dissociative symptoms (depersonalized out-of-body experiences), and the parasympathetic-immobilized freeze response. As an example, when an attack becomes imminent, in the absence of fight-or-flight options, freeze is often combined with analgesia. This defensive reaction is believed to potentially reduce the likelihood of continued attack. If the continued attack is not reduced, the depersonalization (out-of-body experience) or anesthesias minimize the subjective impact.

2. The *sympathetic nervous system* (SNS) is the system of mobilization. It prepares the body for emergency and aspects of fight or flight by increasing cardiac output, stimulating sweat glands, and inhibiting the metabolically costly gastrointestinal system.

3. The *ventral vagal complex*, situated in the nucleus ambiguous of the medulla, is a parasympathetic system that enables rapid engagement and disengagement in the environment by applying a more subtle and flexible gentle braking when needed. By increasing or decreasing this advanced vagal brake, sympathetic activity can be increased or decreased in subtle variations. Therefore, rather than directly engaging the adrenal SNS, which is metabolically more costly and less precise (fine tuned) when engaging the environment, this braking facilitates the subtle sympathetic increases or decreases, enabling the nuanced and more sophisticated aspects of mammalian and, especially, human interactive and affect-regulatory function.

Porges (2001,2011) argues that through stages of phylogeny (the evolution of a species), mammals and especially primates have evolved a functional neural organization that regulates visceral state (internal organs and musculature) in order to support social behavior. Specifically, he proposes a social engagement system that focuses predominantly on the neural regulation of the striated muscles of the face and head, in combination with the specific autonomic functions of the myelinated branch of the *ventral vagus*. As an example, reflect on the nuances of interactions that are noticeable in primates and humans. In contrast to lower mammals (horses, cats, dogs), we are able to discern a remarkable increase in sophisticated changes of facial expression and vocal communication. To be sure, some of these features do exist in dogs, horses, and cats, but at a more subtle (less sophisticated) and less discernible manner.

Social Engagement and the Vagus Nerve

This social engagement system, through control components in the orbitofrontal cortex, regulates brainstem circuitry that controls eyelid opening (visual gaze); facial muscles (emotional expression); middle-ear muscles (extracting the human voice from background noise); laryngeal and pharyngeal muscles (vocalization, prosody, and language); and head-turning muscles (social gesture and orientation). Collectively, these muscles both regulate social engagement and modulate the sensory features (information) of the environment.

Thus, in general, but especially in the context of human development, the neural control of these muscles contributes to the richness of both social expression and social experience. The source of this neural control, the ventral vagus, is located in the nucleus ambiguous of the medulla, providing the source of a socializing and neural inhibitory component of the nervous system. This inhibitory system promotes calm states consistent with the metabolic demands of neural growth and restoration by slowing heart rate, lowering blood pressure, and inhibiting sympathetic activation at the level of the heart.

Aspects of this social engagement system are functional soon after birth and develop rapidly to support communication and attachment with the environment. Hence, as we noted above, when an infant encounters the caregiver's face, the infant will attempt to engage via facial expression and vocalization. Negative states will be signaled by crying and grimacing. Alternatively, a wide-eyed, smiling infant will attempt to elicit positive vocalizations and wide-eyed smiles from the caregiver. Porges (2001) notes that "even in the young infant, the social engagement system expects face-to-face interactions, with contingent facial expressions and vocalizations" (p. 125).

Vagal Inhibition, Sympathetic Arousal, and Emotional Operating Systems

If we pause and reflect on the foregoing, we see yet another layer of evolution's role in affective regulation and attachment.

Recall that the seeking system mediates and motivates us to search for the things we need, crave, and desire. In combination with the mediating sympathetic circuitry noted above, it is the ventral vagal brake that mediates the increase and decrease in vagal tone, which mediates the increase and decrease of sympathetic energy, as needed, without directly engaging the adrenal sympathetic system. Therefore, by default, changes in *parasympathetic braking* are more precise than changes in *sympathetic throttle* function. Hence, the needed incremental change is more finely tuned. To illustrate with another example, changing the amount of air that a fire gets allows for a more graded and precise control of the heat it gives off than does adding or removing the wood that it feeds on. In the same way, the ventral vagal brake is more precise and graded than the sympathetic throttle.

In the panic system, evolution has provided safeguards to assure that parents take care of their offspring, while giving their young and dependent offspring a powerful emotional system to indicate that they are in need of care (as reflected in paniclike crying and other separation calls). In the same manner as in the seeking system, the ventral vagal brake allows for finer-tuned changes to facilitate attachment and its concomitant affective regulation.

In the fear system, which mediates flight and freeze, numerous polyvagal mediations can come into play. In flight, the sympathetic system can be activated for utmost energy usage. In sympathetic hypervigilant freeze, the sympathetic system would still predominate. In parasympathetic freeze, the dorsal vagus would mediate the immobilization and resultant dissociative processes.

In the rage system, maximal adrenal sympathetic arousal would mediate predominantly for as long as the prolonged challenge continues.

Affective Regulation and Cardiac Dominance

Note that despite the fact that the vagus nerve is interconnected with every major organ, muscle, and glandular system, the major organizing center of its function appears to be the heart. Why would that be? Recall that the early developing sympathetic neural circuitry is energy expanding, whereas the later-developing parasympathetic circuitry is energy conserving. Consequently, evolution selected the heart as the central organizer because regulation of the heart determines the availability of metabolic resources required for mobilization (energy expansion) as well as for growth and restoration (energy conservation). For example, cardiac output must be *regulated* in order to remain calm, *mobilized* for fight-or-flight needs, or relatively *immobilized* for avoidance (depersonalization) or feigned death. Accordingly, these structures represent two global and often opposing systems, with the parasympathetic inhibitory system as dominant (by default), under optimal development and/ or circumstance (Porges, 2001; Thayer & Lane, 2009).

The apparent reason for ventral vagal inhibition's role as the default brain state is that it allows for fine and delicate regulation of heart rate, in response to ever-changing environmental demands. If the sophisticated ventral vagal brake is available by default, we can rapidly increase cardiac output by various degrees, without necessarily having to engage the sympathetic adrenal system. This would allow for various modes of mobilization that are not *emergency driven*. If situations do become more emergent, the option is always there to engage full sympathetic arousal. However, the ability to rapidly reengage the ventral vagal brake inhibits sympathetic activity, allowing for a rapid decrease in metabolic output to self-soothe and calm rather than *slamming* on the brake with the dorsal vagus (Porges, 1997, 2001).

Polyvagal Function and Dissolution

Porges (1997) maintains that this phylogenetically based hierarchical response strategy is consistent with the concept of *dissolution* proposed by John Hughlings Jackson (1869/1958), wherein "the higher nervous arrangements inhibit (or control) the lower, and thus, when the higher are suddenly rendered functionless, the lower rise in activity" (as cited in Porges, 2001, p. 132).

Porges (2011) notes that in this phylogenetically structured hierarchy, the most recent circuit associated with social communication, the ventral vagus, is utilized first. If that circuit fails to provide safety, as in extreme danger, or is developmentally unattainable, then the older survival-oriented circuits are recruited sequentially: the SNS first and the dorsal vagus thereafter.

Unfortunately, from a developmental perspective, the oldest, most primitive, circuits develop first, and the most recent circuit develops last, thereby rendering the child most sensitive to postpartum life and, hence, vulnerable to neural insult. The most recent circuit becomes only partially available during the last trimester and is expressed at term (birth), mediated by the brainstem reflexes that enable the coordination of sucking, swallowing, and breathing. By 6 months postpartum, these brainstem reflexes, which become partially connected to cortical processes in the lateral orbitofrontal, provide a biobehavioral pathway through which reciprocal social engagement behavior can calm and soothe the physiological state in both participants of a social dyad (e.g., mother–infant interactions).

Therefore, until the age of approximately 3 years, the caregiver is required to *function as a ventral vagal brake*, given that prior to that age the child's ventral vagus can mediate only attachment functions but not the affect-regulatory roles. We will return to this when we examine neglectful and abusive parenting and the resultant dissolution of affective regulation.

Orbitofrontal Affective Regulation

Recollect that in the second year, the growth and expansion of axons from noradrenergic sites in the lateral orbitofrontal cortex (OFC) to brainstem areas in the medulla allow for the lateral OFC's role in mediating the vagal restraint, noted above, and the subsequent energy-conserving inhibition of sympathetic autonomic arousal. In addition to these orbitomedullary connections, the lateral areas of the OFC also grow and expand into areas of the hypothalamus, which also influence heart function in concert with the medullary/vagal influence.

As we noted above, prior to this development, the loving caregiver's facial features and vocal prosody are *required* to trigger the earlier-forming corticobulbar (brainstem) pathways that recruit the vagal brake, to calm the child. Hence, these final advanced orbitofrontal–vagal connections *complete* the organization of the parasympathetic centers of the OFC, giving the child the ability to *increasingly self-soothe*, adaptively, in the absence of caregiver soothing, without having to resort to primitive (dorsal vagal), pathological self-soothing. By the middle of the second year, these neuropsychobiological advances enable the *automodulation* of hyperactive behaviors and hyper-aroused states.

Left Hemispheric Dorsolateral Development

In the middle of the second year, a major transition in maturation and development ensues. With respect to maturation, as the orbital prefrontal growth spurt concludes, a significant period is initiated for the maturation of the other major prefrontal division, the dorsolateral cortex. This transitional event also represents a shift in growth and expansion from the earlier-maturing right hemisphere to the later-maturing left hemisphere (Schore, 1994). In the transition from the *practicing* period to the rapprochement period, the child's emotional transactions with the mother become more ambivalent as she continues to separate and individuate, propelling her closer to her father.

Returning to anatomy, the maturational growth and expansion of the left dorsolateral cortex into subcortical areas manifests in connections into nonlimbic areas, as opposed to the expansion of the orbitofrontal, which manifests connections into limbic and affect mediating areas. Consequently, Tucker (1992) notes that the early maturation of the right hemisphere is adaptive and consistent with the importance of emotional communication and symbiosis in early life. In the second year, however, the child's increasing motor competence and rapid development of language skills reflect the major transition in brain maturation toward left hemisphere dominance. Hence, this is expressed in the shift from attentional and emotional dependence on the social environment, mediated by the right hemisphere, toward an increasing articulation of cognitive and motor control, and increasing emotional and attentional autonomy, mediated by the increase in left hemispheric development and expansion into subcortical areas.

Thus, the orbitofrontal cortex mediates the executive control of the right hemisphere, whereas the dorsolateral cortex mediates the executive control of the left hemisphere.

Unconscious Memorial and Affective Templates

Returning to the orbitofrontal cortex, it is the experience-dependent maturation of its subcortical and cortical circuits that is responsible for the development of the temperamental dispositions that underlie personality styles. The older child's (and eventually, the adult's) biologically organized emotional core is *biased* toward certain emotional responses that are, by now, driven by the neural templates (emotions, cognitions/beliefs, and memories) of his early attachment experiences (Bechara, Damasio, Tranel, & Damasio, 1997). Hence, present life interpersonal experiences activate the neural maps of earlier childhood. This occurs *unconsciously* and, often, regardless of what is actually occurring, thus biasing our emotional perception of personal interactions (Hugdahl, 1995).

Therefore, the processing of socioaffective stimuli (interpersonal and/or attachment driven) is relayed to the orbitofrontal cortex to be matched against earlier-formed childhood imprinted experiential neural templates, mediating an unconscious *appraisal* of the situation's emotional meaning. Hence, appraisal represents an evaluation of the personal/emotional significance of what is happening in this interpersonal encounter with the environment. Thus, in this process, perceptions of current environmental socioemotional information are computed in relation to the practicing-period-derived paralimbic templates (internal unconscious working models) of our predispositional, affectively-charged interactive memories and representations (Schore, 2003b; Zald & Kim, 1996).

Therefore, in our emotionally significant interpersonal interactions, our *expectations* are derived more from our childhood experiences than from what is actually occurring. As an example, reflect on the differences between casual work relationships and emotionally significant relationships, and notice how work relations are generally uncomplicated and orderly, whereas personal relationships become increasingly complex, less than consciously rational, often confusing, unconsciously driven, and emotionally immediate. This is also in stark contrast to functioning in cognitive domains, which is *conscious* and more present oriented with respect to appraisal and reaction.

Recall that emotional memory and its resultant emotions are nondeclarative, in that emotional memory is derived from experience but is expressed as a change in behavior or emotional state rather than as a recollection. Consequently, we refer to nondeclarative memory and its resultant emotion as *reflexive* and to declarative memory and its resultant recollection as *reflective*. Recollect also that Squire and Kandel (1999) have argued,

> In no small part, by virtue of the unconscious status of these forms of memory . . . arise the dispositions, habits, and preferences that are inaccessible to conscious recollection but that nevertheless are shaped by past events, influence our behavior and mental life, and are an important part of who we are. (p. 193)

If we ask ourselves why evolution has created such a system, we have yet to arrive at a satisfying answer. Remember, that despite its relatively small size, the brain accounts for about 20% of the energy consumed by the entire body. Furthermore, relative to this very high rate of energy consumption, the *additional* energy consumption associated with evoked changes in the brain (processing information from the external world) is remarkably small, often less than 5%. Therefore, the overwhelming majority of the energy utilized by the brain is for our *intrinsic inner reality*, whereas only a small amount is utilized to deal with any aspect of our *outer reality*.

Not surprisingly, we know as clinicians that the majority of emotional problems that befall us, from neuroses to personality disorders to posttraumatic and dissociative disorders, are driven by intrinsic emotional perceptions that are no longer accurately congruent with extrinsic reality. As we have previously noted, it certainly begs the question as to whether our consciousness, intrinsic as it is, *by design*, is indeed adaptive or an evolutionary flaw yet to be tinkered with.

CHAPTER 7

Disorders of Consciousness

Consciousness is something that every child understands, yet scientists and philosophers struggle to explain it. We are all intimately familiar with what it means to be conscious or unconscious as we awaken in the morning, drift off to sleep at night, find our attention drifting or dozing off, briefly, during a lecture, walk through a forest enjoying the beauty; all without having to pay attention to our gait, while engaged in a stimulating discussion. Consciousness provides an essential human quality to our life experience, as we depend on it to organize and prioritize our memories, emotions, and actions. Consequently, when consciousness is impaired or removed, the absence of this seamless organization becomes crippling, bringing us to our knees.

Unraveling the enigma of consciousness, and its impairment and disturbance, has been a thorny road to travel, often littered with confusion and denial. This has been particularly true with regard to our understanding of the effects of psychological neglect and trauma on our biopsychosocial systems.

GLOBAL ALTERATIONS OF CONSCIOUSNESS

Consciousness is alterable by a number of influences: alcohol, drugs, anesthesia, childhood neglect and abuse, traumatic experiences, neural injury, and disease. Therefore, it is by examining how human consciousness is drastically changed by anatomical or functional changes in the brain, as well as considering which changes in brain structure and dynamics do not affect consciousness, that we can better understand both the neural nature of consciousness as well as its disrepair.

Accordingly, we will begin by exploring briefly global alterations of consciousness, such as anesthesia, coma, and vegetative states. This will allow us to examine the impact of these pervasive states of impaired consciousness on the neural systems, noted above. We will examine in detail disorders of consciousness induced by psychic neglect and trauma.

Anesthesia

The most common external manipulation of consciousness is general anesthesia. Consequently, anesthetics can also be used as tools in the study of consciousness, in that they provide a stable reproducible temporary reduction or elimination of consciousness from which comparisons in brain functioning can be made throughout transitions between the conscious and unconscious state, and vice versa.

Anesthetics consist of two main classes: intravenous agents used for induction, such as profolol and ketamine, generally administered together with sedatives such as midazolam and dexedetomidine; and inhaled agents, such as isoflurane, sevoflurane, and desflurane, or the gases xenon and nitrous oxide (Alkire, 2009).

At the cellular level, many anesthetics have mixed effects, but the overall result is a decrease in neural excitability, by either increasing inhibition or decreasing excitation. Regardless of the neurotransmitter mediation, the overall cellular result is *cellular hyperpolarization*. Recall that depolarization increases the cell's ability to generate an action potential and is considered to be excitatory. Conversely, hyperpolarization makes it unlikely that a cell will generate an action potential and is, therefore, considered inhibitory.

At the neuroimaging level, the specific details have been difficult to ascertain. However, the contours of the circuitry involved have been clearer. The case can be made for a common effect of most, if not all, anesthetic agents involving thalamic metabolic blood flow and thalamocortico–corticothalamic (thalamus-to-cortex–cortex-to-thalamus) connectivity (Alkire, 2009). The *details* regarding whether the thalamus is, in effect, switching off the cortex or the cortex is switching off the thalamus are not yet inferable. However, the *contour*, manifested by the thalamocortical circuitry and its impaired overall regional connectivity, is clear. Recall, that it is the thalamocortical circuitry that mediates the binding of the spatial maps of our extrinsic and intrinsic functioning. Recent data (Cotterill, 2001) have suggested that this circuitry should be extended to the lateral cerebellothalamocortical system.

Coma and Vegetative States

Whereas consciousness may grow fainter during certain phases of sleep and be kept at very low levels during general anesthesia, coma and vegetative states are characterized by a loss of consciousness that is difficult and often impossible to reverse.

Coma, an enduring sleeplike state of immobility from which the patient cannot be aroused, represents the *quintessential* form of pathological loss of consciousness (Posner & Plum, 2007). Typically, coma is caused by a suppression of corticothalamic function by drugs, toxins, or internal metabolic pathology. Other causes of coma include head trauma, strokes, or hypoxia (loss of oxygen).

Patients who survive a coma may recover, whereas others enter a vegetative state, in which the eyes reopen, giving the appearance of wakefulness, but their unresponsiveness persists. Postmortem analyses of vegetative patients reveal that the brainstem, hypothalamus, and reticular activation systems remain intact, explaining why these patients look awake. Studies indicate that the vegetative state is due to widespread lesions of the gray matter in the neocortex and thalamus, widespread white matter damage, or bilateral thalamic lesions, especially to the *intralaminar paramedian thalamic* nuclei (Posner & Plum, 2007). Indeed, recovery from vegetative states has been associated with the restoration of functional connectivity between intralaminar thalamic nuclei and prefrontal and cingulate cortices (Laureys et al., 2000).

Recollect that damage to nuclei of the specific thalamocortical system produces only a loss of the particular sensory modality that was mediated by the specific damaged nucleus. However, following damage to nuclei of the nonspecific *intralaminar* thalamocortical system, all perception and, therefore, consciousness ceases. All extrinsic information mediated by the specific circuitry of the system can no longer be perceived or responded to. In essence, as Llinas (2001) describes, "the individual no longer exists, from a cognitive point of view, and although specific sensory inputs to the cortex remain intact, they are completely ignored" (p. 127).

PSYCHOTRAUMATIC ALTERATIONS OF CONSCIOUSNESS

Life is an enduring struggle for people who have been traumatized. Their torment essentially recounts a horrific and anguished past that haunts them, relentlessly. Bessel van der Kolk and Alexander McFarlane (1996) contend that "experiencing trauma is an essential part of being human; history is written in blood" (p. 3). Centuries of wars, famines, pogroms, holocausts, slavery, dictatorship, and colonization have brought every type of horror and abuse into the homes of our ancestors. Some found ways to adapt, but many succumbed to the misery and desolation. Despite humanity's capacity to survive and adapt, traumatic experiences alter biological, psychological, and social equilibrium to such a vast extent that the memory and interpretation of traumas wash over and taint all other experiences, contaminating the present and future (van der Kolk & McFarlane, 1996).

Judith Herman (1992) notes that psychological trauma

> . . . is an affliction of the powerless. At the moment of trauma, the victim is rendered helpless by overwhelming force. When the force is that of nature, we speak of *disasters* [emphasis added]. When the force is that of other human beings, we speak of *atrocities* [emphasis added]. Traumatic events overwhelm the ordinary systems of care that give people a sense of control, connection, and meaning. (p. 33)

Hence, the common denominator of trauma is a feeling of intense fear, helplessness, loss of control, and threat of annihilation (Andreasen, 1985).

Judith Herman (1992) argues that the severity of traumatic events cannot be understood or measured on any single dimension, noting that "simplistic efforts to quantify trauma ultimately lead to meaningless comparisons of horror" (p. 34). Nonetheless, certain circumstances or events likely increase the potential for traumatization, among them physical violation or injury, relational trauma, exposure to extreme violence, or witnessing grotesque death. In all cases, "the salient characteristic of the traumatic event is its power to inspire helplessness and terror" (p. 34).

Trauma and Dissociation

Van der Hart, Nijenhuis, and Steele (2006) note that chronically traumatized people are caught in an appalling dilemma. Unable to process and integrate their painful experiences, they must, nonetheless, go on with a daily life that sometimes continues to include the very people who abused and neglected them. Even if their abusers are no longer present, they must continue to struggle to function adaptively. Consequently, their most expedient option (as conserved by evolution and adapted by humans) is to mentally avoid their unresolved and painful past and present and, as much as possible, try to maintain an internal as well as external *facade of normality*.

The coexistence of and relationship between trauma and dissociative disorders have only recently become clear. Herman (1992) observes that traumatic reactions occur when the option of *action* is lost, rendering the systems of self-defense overwhelmed and disorganized. Components of the systems dedicated to responses to danger, having lost their utility, tend to persist in altered and exaggerated forms long after the danger has ceased. Traumatic events produce lasting impairments in physiological arousal, emotion, cognition, and memory, *severing* these normally integrated functions from each other. Herman argues that in this resultant state of dissociation, memory, affect, and cognition become *disconnected* (unlinked), taking on a life of their own.

Similarly, van der Hart, Nijenhuis, and Steele (2006) argue that dissociation is the key concept to understanding traumatization. They view the spectrum of acute posttraumatic stress disorder (PTSD), depersonalization disorder, dissociative amnesia, dissociative fugue, and dissociative identity disorder (DID) as a spectrum of structural dissociation of the personality (Nijenhuis, van der Hart, & Steele, 2002; van der Hart & Nijenhuis, 1998; van der Hart, Nijenhuis, & Steele, 2006; van der Hart, Nijenhuis, & Steele, 2005; van der Hart, Nijenhuis, Steele, & Brown, 2004). They maintain that a century of studying psychotraumatology has illustrated that traumatized people tend to alternate between intrusive reexperiencing, being detached from, and being unaware of their traumas, as a result of amnesia.

In concert with this shift, the syndrome of psychological difficulties that have been revealed to be frequently associated with histories of protracted and marked interpersonal abuse has been named *complex PTSD* or *disorders of extreme stress, not otherwise specified* (DES/NOS) (Herman, 1992; van der Kolk, Perry, & Herman, 1991). These diagnoses describe the following six clusters of symptoms that are regularly observed in dissociative disorders (van der Kolk, 2001):

1. Alterations in the regulation of affect and impulses, including difficulties in the modulation of anger and self-destructiveness
2. Alterations in attention and consciousness, often leading to amnesias, dissociative episodes, and depersonalizations
3. Alterations in self-perception, such as a chronic sense of guilt, responsibility, and shame
4. Alterations in relationship to others, compromised by the inability to trust and feel intimate
5. Various degrees of physiological disorders and disease processes, which have been described as medically unexplained symptoms
6. Impairment vis-à-vis the integrated functioning of their identity mechanisms

Trauma, Attachment, and Personality

Classen, Pain, Field, and Woods (2006) have argued for the inception of a new diagnostic category, posttraumatic personality disorder (PTPD), to articulate the interrelationship of chronic traumatization, disorganized attachment disorders, dissociative disorders, and borderline personality disorders (BPDs). They note that although complex PTSD, or DES/NOS, is intended to reflect the consequences of chronic traumatization, the domains that they describe are characterized more accurately as a personality disorder, more specifically, a PTPD. They suggest two types of PTPD: one involving organized attachment and the other concerning disorganized attachment, both associated with PTSD.

Classen et al. (2006) propose that PTPD reflects a history of extensive chronic traumatization beginning in childhood. They contend further that "disorganized attachment underlies BPD and, thus, the symptoms characteristic of BPD (affective disturbances, disturbed cognition, impulsivity, primitive defense mechanisms, and intense relational instability) are viewed as pathological adaptations to living with a disorganized attachment pattern" (p. 88). Consequently, PTPD/disorganized designates the comorbidity of BPD and DES/NOS.

Alternatively, these authors argue that chronic child neglect and abuse of children who have experienced a more organized attachment with their parents tend to lead to PTPD/organized. Accordingly, PTPD/organized represents DES/NOS without BPD. They opine further that the sole diagnosis of BPD should be made with individuals who have a disorganized attachment but a less severe history of child abuse.

These researchers posit that understanding the effect of chronic traumatization in the context of either organized or disorganized attachment has specific implications for treatment for further research.

Childhood Trauma and Development

Bessel van der Kolk (2005) and van der Kolk and d'Andrea (2010) argue for the urgent need for a developmentally sensitive interpersonal trauma diagnosis for children, that of developmental trauma disorder. They maintain that the severe and chronic impairments to emotional regulation, impulse control, attention, cognition, dissociation, interpersonal relationships, and relational schemas, resulting from childhood relational neglect and trauma, are best understood as a single, coherent disorder.

Van der Kolk and d'Andrea (2010) note that the numerous clinical expressions of the damage resulting from childhood relational trauma are currently relegated to a "variety of seemingly unrelated comorbidities" such as conduct disorder, attention deficit disorder, phobic anxiety, separation anxiety, and reactive attachment disorder. Hence, the conceptual specificity of developmental trauma disorder, inherently, distinguishes it from the existing symptomatic and comorbid diagnoses that currently prevail. They opine further that

> . . . the continued practice of applying multiple distinct comorbid diagnoses to traumatized children has grave consequences; it defies parsimony, obscures etiological clarity, and runs the danger of relegating treatment and intervention to a small aspect of the child's psychopathology, rather than promoting a comprehensive treatment approach. (p. 61)

These conceptual changes, informed by decades of clinical experience, reflect the impression that trauma and dissociation do, indeed, appear to coexist and are, evidently, driven by similar evolutionarily based biological action systems.

The Evolution of Biological Action Systems

The relationship of posttraumatic and dissociative symptoms to the biological emotional operating systems (Panksepp, 1998), fixed action patterns (Llinas, 2001), functional systems (Fanselow & Lester, 1988), and dispositions (Damasio, 1999, 2010) that were noted above requires further elaboration. For convenience, these systems will be termed "biological action systems" (Nijenhuis et al., 2002). Recall (from Chapter 5) that Panksepp lists six objective neural criteria that define emotional operating systems, frequent action patterns, and dispositions (action systems) in the brain. These criteria are as follows:

1. The underlying circuits must be genetically predetermined and designed to respond unconditionally to stimuli arising from major life-challenging circumstances.
2. These circuits must organize diverse behaviors by activating or inhibiting motor circuits and concurrent autonomic hormonal changes that have proved to be adaptive in the face of such life-challenging circumstances during the evolutionary history of the species.
3. These emotional circuits must change the sensitivities of sensory systems that are relevant to the behavioral sequences that have been aroused.
4. The neural activity of these emotional systems must outlast the precipitating circumstances, indicating their evolutionary stability and consistency over time.
5. These emotional circuits can come under the conditional control of emotionally neutral environmental stimuli, as evidenced by anticipatory drives toward exploration of the environment, seeking warmth and sexual gratification, as well as attachment.
6. These circuits must have reciprocal interactions with the brain mechanisms that elaborate higher decision-making processes and consciousness.

Emotional Action Systems

As we also noted above, Panksepp (1998) designates the following emotional operating systems (action systems) as defined primarily by genetically coded neural circuits that generate well-organized emotional and behavioral sequences, which can be evoked by localized electrical stimulation of these neural circuits in the brain:

1. The seeking system, which mediates interest in and exploration of the environment, food seeking, warmth, and sexual gratification
2. The fear system, which mediates flight or freeze
3. The rage system, which mediates fight.
4. The panic system, which mediates distress vocalization and social attachment

These systems (as described in Chapter 5), therefore, are the basic elements that shape personality. Over the course of evolution, these primitive action systems (fixed action patterns and dispositions) have become linked with higher cortical functions, enabling us to engage in complex action tendencies, including complex relationships (van der Hart, Nijenhuis, and Steele,

2006). Functioning as adults, therefore, involves a profound complexity of biopsychosocial goals (caring for children, socializing, competing, loving and protecting, and exploring our inner and outer worlds). Meeting these goals involves a deep integration of these action systems. We will return to this.

Action Systems, Trauma, and Dissociation

Van der Hart, Nijenhuis, and Steele (2006) argue that traumatic and dissociative symptoms involve a particular organization of the psychobiological systems that constitute the personality or the self. Consequently, this organization is neither arbitrary nor coincidental but is mediated by well-defined, evolutionarily conserved neural systems. Accordingly, they view posttraumatic and dissociative symptoms as driven by structural dissociation of the personality. Therefore, dissociative phenomena are driven not just by mental actions, such as experiencing sensations or affects, but rather by the two major *categories* of biological action systems that appear to constitute the self.

Approach and Avoidance

Recall that one category involves neural systems that are principally geared to the *approach* toward attractive stimuli in daily life, such as attaching to one's mother and father, eating, drinking, playing with friends, or being sexual. The other category of neural systems mediates the *avoidance* or escape from noxious, aversive, or threatening stimuli. Echoing Panksepp's (1998) formulations, van der Hart et al. (2006) note,

> The evolutionary purpose of these systems is to help us distinguish between helpful and harmful experiences, and to generate the best adaptive responses to current life circumstances. These situations encompass our interoceptive and exteroceptive worlds, our internal and external environment, as we perceive them. We refer to these psychobiological systems as *action systems*, because each involves particular innate propensities to act in a goal directed manner. (p. 3)

Thus, these action tendencies involve adaptations to environmental challenges, both *appetitive* and *aversive*. Each tendency entails a range of mental and behavioral actions. Consequently, these action systems help us to behave, think, feel, and perceive in particular and specific ways that are protective and adaptive. Hence, we feel, think, perceive, and behave in one manner when we are hungry, rather differently when we are curious, and yet again differently when threatened (Damasio, 2010; van der Hart, Nijenhuis, and Steele, 2006).

Systemic Organization

In order to systematize the varied symptom clusters and syndromes of traumatic and dissociative disorders, their organization is required vis-à-vis the phenomenological aspects of *reexperiencing trauma* versus *detachment from trauma* and their relationship to the action systems that mediate them. For example, reexperiencing trauma is associated with the inborn and evolutionarily derived defensive systems of fear and rage that are evoked by severe threat. As complex action systems, they encompass various subsystems, such as flight, freeze, and fight. Therefore, when stimulated, the neural circuitry of the fear system enables us to run away. It can also provoke a freeze response in us. This response can be neurally sympathetic in nature, leading to a hyperaroused stillness (reducing the possibility of attack or destruction), or parasympathetic in nature, leading to a tonic immobility and possible analgesia (reducing the pain of an imminent attack or destruction). The parasympathetic nature of this neural system has often been described as dissociative fugue states, depersonalization (out-of-body experiences), and numbness. The circuitry mediating the rage system is aroused by frustration and attempts to curtail our freedom of action. Consequently, it not only allows us to defend ourselves aggressively but also energizes us when irritated or restrained.

Detachment from trauma is associated with the action systems of seeking and panic, which control functions in daily life (for example, exploration of the environment and energy control), and the ones that are dedicated to survival of the species (reproduction and attachment to and caring for offspring; Nijenhuis et al., 2002; van der Hart, Nijenhuis, and Steele, 2006). In addition, these action systems will also be reviewed in reference to the organizing constructs of primary, secondary, and tertiary dissociation (Nijenhuis et al., 2002; van der Hart, van der Kolk, & Boon, 1996; van der Kolk, van der Hart, & Marmar, 1996; van der Hart, Nijenhuis, and Steele, 2006).

The Nature of Dissociation

As we have already noted, dissociation appears to be key to understanding trauma-induced disorders of consciousness. Van der Hart, Nijenhuis, and Steele (2006) note that we have not come easily to this appreciation, largely because many concepts in the trauma field require clarification, dissociation chief among them. Indeed, defining what dissociation is, or is not, is one can of worms in our field, and its causes an even larger one.

Although the focus of this chapter is pathological, trauma-induced dissociation, it nonetheless begs the question as to whether the various phenomenological manifestations of dissociation are *always* pathological in nature. The answer to this question pertains to two areas of great import: the nature of the human mind and the *self* and its implications for treatment (i.e., does this symptom need to be removed or terminated owing to its pathology, or does it just need to be modified and returned to its normative adaptive level)? To put it another way, if the true normative nature of the self is to be singular and monolithic, then the implications for integration in treatment would be to facilitate the fusion of all self states into one. On the other hand, if the multiplicity of the self is inherently normative, then the implications for integration in treatment would be to facilitate trauma resolution and integrated adaptive function within the inherent normative multiself structure. We will return to this.

Butler (2006) notes that although the literature corresponding to the study of dissociation is concerned primarily with pathology, most dissociative experiences are not pathological, wherein a large proportion of the stream of consciousness is taken up with normative dissociative experiences, such as daydreaming, fantasy, and absorption. There certainly appears to be agreement in our field that dissociative symptoms such as derealization, depersonalization, and fugue states appear to be pathological in origin and nature. The greatest polarity in agreement, however, appears to be with respect to the nature of the multiplicity of the self, specifically, with respect to the formation of self states or ego states.

The Description of Dissociation

Dissociation has been described in the literature as a process, an intrapsychic structure, a psychological defense, a deficit, and an array of other symptoms (van der Hart, Nijenhuis, and Steele, 2006). In the past decade, theoretical and technical writings have centered their ideas around the central point, wherein dissociation is seen as a division of the personality. Specifically, Janet's (1907) definition has been returned to the forefront, in which dissociation is viewed as a division among "systems of ideas and functions that constitute the personality" (p. 332).

Primary Dissociation

As defined by van der Hart, van der Kolk, and Boon (1996) and van der Kolk, van der Hart, and Marmar (1996), primary dissociation refers to the inability to integrate the totality of a traumatic event into consciousness, thereby causing the intrusion into awareness of fragmented traumatic memories, primarily in sensory form. These intrusive sensory fragments tend to be visual, olfactory, auditory, kinesthetic, or visceral. Primary dissociation, therefore, is characteristic of type I PTSD, in which the most dramatic symptoms are expressions of associated traumatic memories, such as intrusive recollections, nightmares, and flashbacks.

These phenomenological responses are often associated with psychophysiological arousal, as evidenced by increased heart rate and electrical skin conductance (Frewen & Lanius, 2006; Orr, McNally, & Rosen, 2004). Van der Kolk, van der Hart, and Marmar (1996) maintain that "this fragmentation is accompanied by ego states that are distinct from the normal state of consciousness" (p. 307). In a more recent conceptualization, called *primary structural dissociation of the personality*, these ego states have been designated as the "apparently normal part" of the personality (ANP) and the "emotional part" of the personality (EP), to designate an aspect of the adult ego state or self and the other dissociated ego states, respectively (Nijenhuis, van der Hart, & Steele, 2002; Steele, van der Hart, & Nijenhuis, 2001). Van der Hart, Nijenhuis, and Steele (2006) argue that the division of the personality results from trauma, noting that "even though dissociative parts have a sense of self, no matter how rudimentary, they are not separate entities, but rather are different, more or less divided psychobiological systems that are not sufficiently cohesive or coordinated within an individual's personality" (p. 30).

Secondary Dissociation

Van der Hart, van der Kolk, and Boon (1996) and van der Kolk, van der Hart, and Marmar (1996) observe that once an individual is in a traumatic (dissociated) state of mind, further disintegration of personal experience can occur. Derealization and depersonalization tend to manifest: People report experiences of leaving their body at the moment of the trauma and observing the trauma from a distance. Therefore, secondary dissociation allows individuals to observe their traumatic experience as spectators and to limit their pain and distress.

Phenomenologically, this produces increased fragmentation and dissociated ego states. Steele et al. (2001) note that in secondary structural dissociation of the personality, this increase in fragmentation is observed in increased divisions of the EPs. Consequently, the increase in ego states (EPs) is seen as trauma driven and, therefore, pathological in nature. Diagnostically, this constellation tends to produce the conditions of complex PTSD, DES/NOS, depersonalization disorders, dissociative amnesia, and dissociative fugue.

Tertiary Dissociation

Van der Hart, van der Kolk, and Boon (1996) and van der Kolk, van der Hart, and Marmar (1996) opine that tertiary dissociation results from the development of "distinct ego states that contain the traumatic experience, consisting of complex identities with distinct cognitive, affective and behavioral patterns" (p. 308). Phenomenologically, this produces severely chaotic and profoundly dissociated alter identities, often with little or no consciousness of each other. Nijenhuis et al. (2002) note that in addition to increased divisions of the EPs, tertiary structural dissociation of the personality also produces further divisions of the ANPs. Diagnostically, this constellation tends to produce the condition of DID. Again, the increase in ego states (ANPs and EPs) is seen as trauma driven and, therefore, pathological in nature.

Developmental Lines of the Personality

Throughout psychiatry's and psychology's history, there has also been a parallel line of thought that has viewed dissociation as a normative *developmental line* of the personality. Prior to Anna Freud's (1936, 1963) conceptualization of developmental lines, the presence of defense mechanisms and anxiety, for example, were viewed solely as pathological manifestations. In her initial writings on defense mechanisms (1936), she first suggested a defense mechanism (sublimation) that was not pathological. Anna Freud's ensuing writings and those of Renee Spitz, Heinz Hartmann, Ernst Kris, and Rudolph Loewenstein ushered in ego psychology and the initial examinations of normative/ adaptive, rather than just pathological, development.

Consequently, defense mechanisms and anxiety were seen as serial progressions in distinct psychic sectors, with continuity and cumulative character (Spitz, 1965). In other words, they existed on a continuum, ranging from normative and adaptive to conflicted and pathological. Therefore, defenses and anxiety were now viewed on the same continuum as psychosexual maturation, drive taming, object relations, adaptive function, identity formation, and internalization. Initially, this change in thinking was painfully revolutionary, shattering the mainstream assumptions of psychic functioning.

Dissociation as a Developmental Line

Inspired by the revolution of ego psychology, a number of clinicians began to examine dissociation in a similar vein. Consequently, as in the other developmental lines, they began to suggest that dissociation, as manifested by multiplicity of the self, be viewed as a dynamic continuum, from healthy/adaptive to pathological, and present, at some level, in all diagnostic categories.

Jacob Moreno (1934, 1943) argued that the mind operated on two levels. One level reflected a pluralistic dimension, manifested by an aggregate or multiplicity of inner roles. These roles were seen to be mediated by distinct and different inner psychic structures. The other level, the meta-role, was seen to consist of the mediation of a unifying function, with respect to the multiplicity of inner roles: a sort of chairman of the inner committee.

Paul Federn (1943, 1947, 1952) posited that normally as well as pathologically, ego states are repressed—successfully in "normal" people and unsuccessfully in "neurotics and psychopaths." He viewed ego states as organized entities of the ego, writing, "I conceive of the ego as not merely the sum of all functions, but as the cathexis (energy) which unites the aggregate into a new mental unity" (1952, p. 185).

John Watkins (1949) described the treatment of an army officer with a phobia of the dark, noting that the successful resolution of the treatment involved more than one ego entity. He wrote further that in contrast to true multiple personality disorders, the two subpersonalities did not emerge spontaneously but could be activated hypnotically. Watkins viewed this experience as "our first direct acquaintance with those covertly segmented personality structures we, now, call ego states" (Watkins & Watkins, 1997, p. ix).

Eric Berne (1957a, 1957b, 1961) extended psychodynamic thought with his elaboration and application of Federn's concept of subdivisions of the mind, predating many of the ideas of Mahler, Kohut, Kernberg, and Watkins and Watkins. He described the states of the ego, phenomenologically, "as a coherent system of feelings related to a given subject, and operationally as a set of coherent behavioral patterns; or pragmatically, as a system of feelings which motivates a related set of behavioral patterns" (1961, p. 17).

John Watkins and Helen Watkins (Watkins, 1978; Watkins & Johnson, 1982; Watkins & Watkins, 1997), drawing from the ideas of Janet, Breuer and Freud, Reik, Federn, and Berne and from the implicit allusions to personality multiplicity in the writings of Fairbairn, Ferenczi, Glover, Guntrip, Searles, Sullivan, and Winnicott, proposed that the self was comprised of ego states, which they defined as "an organized system of behavior and experience whose elements are bound together by some common principle and are separated from other such states by a boundary that is more or less permeable" (Watkins & Watkins, 1997, p. 25). They viewed the formation of ego states on a developmental continuum, theorizing that personality was segmented into self states as a result of normal differentiation, introjection, or trauma (Watkins, 1978; Watkins & Watkins, 1997).

Psychoanalytically oriented developmental infant studies (Beebe & Lachmann, 1992; Emde, Gaensbaure, & Harmon, 1976; Sander, 1977; Stern, 1985; Wolff, 1987) began to suggest that the psyche does not start as an integrated whole but is unitary in origin: a mental structure that begins and continues as a multiplicity of self states that maturationally attain a *feeling* of coherence that *overrides* the awareness of discontinuity. This was seen to lead to the experience of cohesion and a sense of one self (Bromberg, 1994, 1998a). Much of this was spurred on by the writings of Ferenczi (1930), Glover (1932), Sullivan (1940), Fairbairn (1944, 1952), Winnicott (1965), Searles (1977), and Lampl-de-Groot (1981), each of whom, either implicitly or explicitly, accorded the phenomenon of multiplicity of the self to be important in their work.

Michael Gazzaniga and Joseph LeDoux (1978), renowned for their split-brain research, noted that research and clinical observations (Gazzaniga, LeDoux, & Wilson, 1977; Gazzaniga, 1970, 1976) indicate that normatively in people, there may well exist a variety of separate memory banks, each inherently coherent, organized, logical, and with its own set of values. These memory banks do not necessarily communicate with one another inside the brain. They note further that these data require us to consider the possibility that multiple selves exist, each of which can control behavior at various moments in time.

Robert Putnam (1988), then director of the Dissociative Disorder Research Unit of the National Institutes for Mental Health, explored "nonlinear state changes" as a developmental paradigm, stating that, "states appear to be the fundamental unit of organization of consciousness and are detectable from the first moments following birth . . . They are self-organizing and self-stabilizing structures of behavior" (p. 25).

Phillip Bromberg (1998b) argued that "self-experience originates in relatively unlinked self states, each coherent in its own right. . . . The experience of being a unitary self is an acquired, developmentally adaptive, *illusion* [emphasis added] (p. 273).

Richard Schwartz (1995) also articulated a multidimensional view of the personality, combining aspects of family systems theory and the multiplicity of the self. Hence, his internal family systems model views consciousness as made up of various "parts" or subpersonalities, each with its own perspective, interests, memories, and viewpoint. The internal family systems model divides these parts into three types—managers, exiles, and firefighters.

Ramachandran (1995) and Ramachandran and Blakeslee (1998), observed that when confronted with an anomaly or discrepancy, the coping styles of the two cerebral hemispheres are fundamentally different. The left hemisphere tends to smooth over these discrepancies by engaging in denials, confabulations, rationalizations, and even delusions, whereas the right hemisphere appears to be the reality-checking mechanism, more anchored in the truth. Regarding the structure of personality, Ramachandran and Blakeslee maintain that the "*self*" may, indeed, be a useful biological construct based on specific brain mechanisms; a sort of organizing principle that allows us to function more effectively by imposing coherence, continuity and stability on the personality" (p. 272). They opine further that various parts of the brain create a useful representation of the external world and generate the *illusion* of a coherent and monolithic self that endures in space and time.

Joseph LeDoux (2003), an eminent neuroscientist, argues,

> In spite of the long tradition of emphasis on the self as a conscious entity in philosophy and psychology, there is a growing interest in a broader view of the self, one that recognizes the multiplicity of the self and emphasizes distinctions between different aspects of the self, especially conscious and non-conscious aspects. (p. 296)

Michael Gazzaniga and his associates (Gazzaniga, 1989, 1998, 2000; Gazzaniga & LeDoux, 1978; Turk et al., 2002; Turk, Heatherton, Macrae, Kelly, & Gazzaniga, 2003) explored the mechanisms by which the brain creates a unified sense of self. Echoing the work of Ramachandran, they note that split-brain research has identified different cognitive processing styles for the two cerebral hemispheres. The right hemisphere appears to process what it receives and no more, whereas the left hemisphere appears to make elaborations, associations, and searches for logical patterns in the material, even when none are present.

Gazzaniga (2000) has argued that this difference in processing style between the two hemispheres is adaptive and represents an underlying role for the left hemisphere in the generation of a unified consciousness experience. Turk, Heatherton, Macrae, et al. (2003) posit, from the studies mentioned above and many others, the existence of an "interpreter" module in the left hemisphere whose purpose is to unify the multiplicity of experience and function into a single self-constituting narrative. They write, "this interpretive function of the left hemisphere takes available information from a distributed self-processing network and creates a unified sense of self from this input" (p. 76).

Hence, in many of the schools of human behavior theory, psychological and neurobiological, there appears to be an increasingly palpable shift with regard to the understanding of the human mind—a shift from the monolithic view of the self (and its inherent clinical implications) to one of the self as decentered and the mind as a "configuration of shifting, nonlinear, discontinuous states of consciousness, in an ongoing dialectic with the *healthy illusion of unitary selfhood* [emphasis added]" (Bromberg, 1998b, p. 270).

Reconciling Conflicting Views of Dissociation

So, if dissociation is the key concept to understanding traumatization, and acute PTSD, depersonalization disorder, dissociative amnesia, dissociative fugue, and DID constitute a spectrum of structural dissociation of the personality, how do we reconcile these phenomena with these two diametrically opposed views of dissociation?

Recall that traumatic and dissociative symptoms involve a particular organization of the psychobiological systems that constitute the personality or the self and that this organization is mediated by well-defined, evolutionarily conserved neural systems. As we shall see, neither view of dissociation impacts these relationships, differentially. Consequently, the only other variable left to reconcile is how to interpret the view that posttraumatic and dissociative symptoms are driven by structural dissociation. How, then, do we define structural dissociation of the personality?

Fortunately, the solution to this dilemma is not as difficult as it may appear. If one subscribes to the position that the multiplicity of the self results solely from pathology, then the creation of self states, ego states, ANPs, and EPs is viewed as the manifestation of structural dissociation. On the other hand, if one subscribes to the position that the multiplicity of the self is normative and manifested on a dynamic continuum, from adaptive to pathological, then structural dissociation is viewed as the process that *impairs* the normally *adaptive* functioning of self-multiplicity, thereby mediating the phenomenon of pathologically functioning ego states (EPs and ANPs) and alter-identities (alters).

The Neurobiology of Primary Dissociation

In its primary form, this dissociation is conceptualized as between the defensive action systems on the one hand and the action systems that involve managing daily life and survival of the species on the other (Nijenhuis et al., 2002). Symptoms, in general, tend to revolve around hyperarousal and intrusion of memories, sensations, or flashbacks, in fragmented form.

Pathophysiology

As a traumatic event ensues, the amygdala sounds the alarm and sends urgent messages to every major part of the brain. It triggers the secretion of the body's fight-or-flight hormones, and the hypothalamus is signaled to produce corticotrophin-releasing factor (CRF). It mobilizes the cerebellum for movement and signals the medulla to activate the cardiovascular system, the muscles, and other systems. Other circuits signal the locus coeruleus for the secretion of norepinephrine to heighten the reactivity of the brain centers, suffusing the brainstem, limbic system, and neocortex. The hippocampus is signaled for the release of dopamine to allow for the riveting of attention (Goleman, 1995; van der Kolk, 1994). In most cases, the traumatic event wanes, and the systems return to baseline.

If the traumatic response continues unabated, the feelings of loss of control and helplessness continue. The brain undergoes allostatic reequilibration, an uncontrolled continuation of the physiological equilibrium designed by evolution for fight or flight but now happening in the absence of traumatic stimuli. This produces the state that we know as PTSD. The locus coeruleus becomes hyperactive, secreting extra-large doses of norepinephrine in situations that hold no danger but are somehow reminiscent of the trauma. Consequently, sensitization geared toward the sharpening of defensive reflexes, in preparation for fight, withdrawal, or escape, is invoked in situations where the danger no longer exists. As a result, symptoms of hyperarousal, hyperstartle, and hypervigilance ensue.

The hypothalamus becomes hyperactive, continuing to secrete CRF, alerting the body to an emergency that is not there. In contrast to other acute and chronic stress disorders, including major depressive disorders, which have evidenced increased CRF and cortisol levels, cortisol studies (when properly done) of PTSD have consistently shown depressed cortisol levels. We will return to this.

Amygdaloid hyperactive functioning impairs hippocampal processes. Recall from Chapter 4 that in the absence of hippocampal–temporal memorial mediation, persons with PTSD are often unable to differentiate past from present, often finding themselves experientially back in the past. In the absence of hippocampal contextual mediation, traumatized people are often unable to differentiate dangerous situations from nondangerous ones (i.e., the bear in the book, or the bear in my backyard?). Consequently, they either perceive danger when there is none or, conversely, are unable to identify danger when it is present, often putting themselves in harm's way.

The aroused amygdala also signals opioid centers in the cortex to release endorphins. This triggers numbing and anhedonia (van der Kolk, 1994). In effect, the neocortex is taken out of the loop. The frontal cortices are unable to shut the emergency systems down.

This massive secretion of neurohormones mediates the long-term potentiation and, thus, the overconsolidation of traumatic memories (van der Kolk, 1996a). Consequently, the capacity to access relevant memories becomes impaired, leading to an increased tendency toward accessing traumatic memories at the expense of others. As a result, physiological arousal triggers trauma-related memories, and trauma-related memories trigger further arousal. This cycling of remembering and arousal causes a rerelease of stress neurohormones, further rekindling the strength of the memory. Bessel van der Kolk notes that these powerful traumatic memories "attract all associations to themselves, and sap current life of its significance" (p. 229). Similarly, Pierre Janet (1919/1925) observed,

> All the famous moralists of olden days drew attention to the way in which certain events would leave indelible and distressing memories—memories to which the sufferer was continually returning, and by which he was tormented by day and night. (p. 589)

Action Systems and Primary Structural Dissociation

Therefore, rather than processing traumatic memories in a nonaroused and integrated manner (contextually and temporally), primary dissociative responses in PTSD involve the emotional and phenomenological reliving of traumatic memories as if they are occurring at the moment of recall. From a neurocognitive perspective, the struggle of biological action systems manifests in conscious or unconscious phobic avoidance of stimuli or cues related to the trauma versus remembering and reliving the traumatic event.

Van der Hart, Nijenhuis, and Steele (2006) maintain that the primary structural dissociation of PTSD produces a dissociated self state or EP that is, essentially, mediated by the inborn and evolutionarily derived defensive action systems of fear *or* rage. As complex action systems, they encompass various subsystems, such as flight, freeze, and fight. The adult self or ANP appears to be more engaged in everyday life. Its function in the structural dissociation of PTSD is detachment from trauma and associated with the action systems of seeking and panic, which control functions in daily life (such as exploration of the environment and energy control), and the ones that are dedicated to survival of the species (reproduction, attachment, and care for offspring).

The adult self or ANP was considered by Myers (1940) and van der Hart et al. (2006) as "apparently normal" because in order to detach from the trauma and continue functioning, it utilizes degrees of amnesia for the trauma, as well as intermittent anesthesia of various sensory modalities, and emotional constriction (Nijenhuis et al., 2002). Therefore, this model maintains that the primary structural dissociation of PTSD produces a dissociated traumatized self or EP characterized by animal defenselike reactions, wherein EPs are fixated on threat cues. Simultaneously, the adult self or ANP is characterized by avoidance of these threat cues.

According to van der Hart, Nijenhuis, and Steele in their various writings, PTSD is viewed as a manifestation of dissociation because EPs and ANPs have different psychobiological stress responses that do not integrate to either unconditional or conditional threat-related stimuli. In other words, neither responds to stimuli in the environment appropriately, nor are they able to integrally balance or regulate each other adaptively.

Essentially, regardless of one's heuristic explanation of the phenomenon of dissociation and self-multiplicity, type I PTSD is considered to be a dissociative disorder because the neurobiological action systems of seeking and panic are dissociated from (not integrated with) the systems of fear and rage. Van der Hart et al. (2006) argue that whereas evolution has given us neural systems that mediate exploration and attachment, and for survival under threat, we are not able to engage both *simultaneously* with any ease. Thus, when both are deemed necessary, a rigid division of the personality ensues to deal with these very discrepant goals and their related actions. As a result, this level of dissociation impairs the ability to smoothly shift through the gears (neural action systems) of exploration of the environment, energy control, sexual function, attachment, caring for offspring, anxiety, and anger.

Think of it: Functioning adaptively requires the integration of all these action systems. Normally, at any given moment of the day, anxiety and anger can be part and parcel of exploration, sexual gratification, attachment, and caring for offspring. Consequently, amnesia, intermittent anesthesia of various sensory modalities, and emotional constriction on the one hand and intrusive recollections and flashbacks on the other hand create maladaptive neural mapping, thereby precluding one's capacity to assimilate new experiences, as if one's personality is frozen at a certain point and cannot expand any more by the addition or assimilation of new elements or experiences. Hence, this rigid division of neural systems creates this form of trauma-induced structural dissociation of the personality or self, a deficiency in the cohesiveness and flexibility of these evolutionarily conserved neural systems.

Temporal Binding and Primary Structural Dissociation

In type I PTSD (primary structural dissociation), manifested by hyperarousal, flashbacks, and reliving, one of the most compelling and informative findings has been the reduced activation of the thalamus (Bremner, Staib, & Kaloupek, 1999; Lanius, Williamson, & Densmore, 2001; Lanius, Williamson, & Hopper, 2003; Liberzon, Taylor, & Amdur, 1999). Lanius, Bluhm, and Lanius (2007) note that this has by no means been consistent across all studies. However, they argue that possible factors that may have accounted for such discrepancies include the following: differences in response variables measured in different studies (i.e., metabolism, regional cerebral blood flow, and blood oxygenation); variability in scanner resolution; and variability in the details of the experimental paradigms [i.e., comorbidity and/or the presence of complex (secondary or tertiary dissociation) PTSD].

Recollect that the nonspecific circuitry of the thalamus is required to achieve temporal binding, that is, to place the representation of specific external sensory images, into one's internal subjective context. Therefore, the thalamocortical circuitry works as a closed system, a neural scaffolding that synchronously relates the sensorily referred properties of the external world to internally generated associations, emotions, motivations, and memories. Consequently, as Llinas (2001) argues, "this temporally coherent event that binds, in the time domain, the fractured components of external and internal reality into a single integrated construct is what we call the *self*" (p. 126).

Therefore, the findings of reduced thalamic activation are likely to indicate impaired temporal binding (temporal mapping). If so, this impairment would be consistent with the following: (a) failure in somatosensory integration, manifested by fragmentation with respect to olfactory memories, auditory memories, gustatory (taste) memories, visual flashbacks, and disturbing kinesthetic (bodily) sensations; (b) failure in cognitive integration, manifested by distorted self-blame and shame; (c) memory fragmentation, manifested by overconsolidated episodic memory coupled with impaired semantic memory, as well as temporal and contextual impairments; (d) failure in emotional function and integration, manifested by hyperarousal and hypervigilance; and (e) failure to integrate the biological action systems in an adaptive manner. In addition, impaired temporal binding could very well impact neural linkage (spatial mapping), leading to the earlier findings of reduced left dorsolateral prefrontal and anterior cingulate activation.

Furthermore, regardless of one's view regarding the origin and nature of internal self states, their function and/or malfunction must also be a product of temporal binding. Ostensibly, then, integrated functioning at *any* level requires, at the basic core, the temporal binding of neural spatial maps into coherent temporal maps.

The Neurobiology of Secondary Dissociation

In contrast to primary dissociation, which emphasizes sensations of reliving traumatic memories, van der Kolk, van der Hart, and Marmar (1996) define secondary dissociation as the mental "leaving" of the body and observing the trauma from a distance. They stress that this manner of psychological distancing of one's conscious awareness limits pain and "puts people out of touch with the feelings and emotions related to the trauma . . . it anesthetizes them" (p. 308). Frewen and Lanius (2006) note that these symptoms are not diagnostic indicators of type I PTSD but rather, of depersonalization disorders. Other diagnostic categories inherent in this group would be dissociative fugue and DD/NOS.

Van der Kolk, van der Hart, and Marmar (1996) note that adults who experience secondary dissociative peritraumatic symptoms may be more likely to have experienced childhood or adolescent traumatic events or abuse and manifest, therefore, poorer psychological adjustment and identity formation, and more vulnerable personality structures.

Secondary Dissociation as a Developmental Disorder

As we noted above, van der Kolk (2005) and van der Kolk and d'Andrea (2010) have argued for a developmentally sensitive interpersonal trauma diagnosis for children: developmental trauma disorder. They maintain that the severe and chronic impairments to emotional regulation, impulse control, attention, cognition, dissociation, interpersonal relationships, and relational schemas, resulting from childhood relational neglect and trauma, are best understood as a developmental disorder.

Consequently, understanding the neural mechanisms of secondary dissociation requires an appreciation of the neural mechanisms of normative human development. Accordingly, as was noted in the previous section on primary dissociation, an essential principle of the developmental psychopathology perspective is that *atypical* pathological development can be understood only in the context of *typical* development, and so the following focus is on underlying mechanisms common to both.

Genesis and Pathophysiology of Secondary Dissociation

In stark contrast to the biopsychosocial environment described in the previous chapter, in severe attachment pathologies, the developing infant or toddler is repeatedly exposed to the ambient cumulative trauma that emanates from an interactive dysregulating context with a misattuned caregiver. The abusive and/or neglectful caregiver not only plays and interacts less with the child but also tends to induce traumatic states of enduring negative affect. Often, this caregiver is emotionally inaccessible and tends to react to the child's expression of emotion and stress inappropriately and/or with rejection. The outcome is minimal or unpredictable participation in the various types of needed arousal regulating processes.

Parental Dysregulation

Rather than modulating their infant's nervous system, such caregivers induce extreme levels of aversive *stimulation* and arousal, either too high, as in *abuse*, or too low, as in *neglect*. This lack of interactive repair maintains the infant's intense negative emotion for long periods. Such affective states contribute to severe alterations in the biochemistry of the child's brain, precluding the proper development of the neuroregulatory circuitry noted above. Recall that the developing brain (unable as yet to self-regulate) can do so properly only in the relational context of another brain that functions as a regulator. Hence, early abuse and/or neglect impact the developing brain. There is extensive evidence that trauma or neglect, early in life, impairs the neural development of the capacities of maintaining adaptive interpersonal relationships (adult or parental), regulating emotion, and coping with stressful stimuli. We will return to this.

Relational Trauma

Childhood trauma can obviously be inflicted from the physical or interpersonal environments. Schore (2003a) and many others have argued that social stressors are *far more detrimental* than nonsocial aversive stimuli, referring to them as *relational trauma*. He notes further that given that such trauma is typically ambient, the stress inherent in ongoing relational trauma is therefore not single-event, or even multiple-event, but *cumulative and ongoing*. Given, as we have already seen, that attachment is the neural regulator that facilitates the proper neural chemistry that promotes the developing brain's growth, early relational trauma has "both immediate and long-term effects, including the generation of risk for later-forming psychiatric disorders" (p. 182).

Dysregulation and Neural Templates

These early dysregulating experiences trigger chaotic alterations in the maturation of the ventral sympathetic orbitofrontal circuitry. Recall that this circuitry mediates aspects of our attachment (panic system) and is centrally involved in our capacity to explore and adapt to our environment and in the organization of new learning (seeking system). Schore (2003a) notes that early relational trauma alters the development of areas of the right hemisphere that are dominant not only for attachment functions but also for the mediation and storage of a working model of attachment relationships, setting the template for future coping styles and relationships. Thus, the affective and relational attachment instability that characterizes dissociative and borderline personality disorders often has its genesis in this pathological neural altering of maturation and development.

In this environment of relational trauma and/or neglect, the caregiver, in addition to dysregulating the infant, is often not available afterward for any repair or reregulating, leaving the infant for long periods in a profoundly disruptive psychobiological state that is beyond his immature nervous system. In studies of neglect, Tronick and Weinberg (1997) note,

When infants are not in homeostatic balance or are emotionally dysregulated (e.g., they are distressed), they are at the mercy of these states. Until these states are brought under control, infants must devote all their regulatory resources to reorganizing them. While infants are doing that, they can do nothing else. (p. 56)

Consequently, infants and children who experience chronic trauma and dysregulation are denied the opportunity for the necessary socioemotional learning during these critical periods of right brain maturation and development.

Recall that regulated affective interactions with a familiar, predictable primary caregiver create not only a sense of safety but also, more important, a *positively charged curiosity* that fuels the burgeoning self's exploration of novel socioemotional and physical environments. Moreover, this ability is a *quintessential marker* of adaptive infant mental health. Hence, as Schore (2003a) notes, "there is a pernicious long-term consequence of relational trauma—an enduring deficit at later points of the life-span in the individual's capacity to assimilate novel (and thus stressful) emotional experiences" (p. 187).

At the beginning of the 20th century, Pierre Janet (1911) argued the following:

All traumatized patients seem to have the evolution of their lives checked; they are attached to an insurmountable object. Unable to integrate traumatic memories, they seem to have lost their capacity to assimilate new experiences as well. It is . . . as if their personality development has stopped at a certain point, and cannot enlarge any more by the addition of new elements. (p. 532, as cited in Schore (2003a), p. 187)

Hence, these traumatic and chronically dysregulated *states*, if maintained and not reregulated, eventually become *traits*, constituting the scaffolding of intrapsychic and interpersonal functioning. We will return to this.

Vagal Consequences

In optimal contexts, both the amygdala and the orbitofrontal cortex (OFC) have direct connections with the lateral hypothalamus, an area known to activate parasympathetic responses through interconnections with the vagus nerve, in the medulla. Recollect that prior to the complete development of the OFC, the loving caregiver's facial features and vocal prosody are *required* to trigger the earlier forming corticobulbar (brainstem) pathways that recruit the ventral vagal brake to calm the child. Hence, these final advanced orbitofrontal–vagal connections, not developed until the middle of the second year, are required to complete the organization of the parasympathetic centers of the OFC, giving the child the ability to *increasingly self-soothe* adaptively in the absence of caregiver soothing, without having to resort to primitive (dorsal vagal), pathological self-soothing.

Dorsal Vagal Regulation

However, because this pathological growth-inhibiting environment generates prolonged levels of negative emotion in the infant, for self-protective purposes, the infant, having made all attempts possible to engage the caregiver in soothing and emotional regulation, withdraws and severely restricts overt expressions of attachment needs for dyadic regulation. Neurologically, the only option available is for the child to engage the primitive dorsal vagus. The child thus significantly reduces the output of his or her emotion-processing, limbic-centered attachment system. So, for defensive functions, the child shifts from interactive, attachment-mediated, regulatory modes into long-enduring, less complex and primitive self-soothing modes. This sets the stage for primitive autoregulation and for the habitual use of dorsal vagal-mediated dissociation. Indeed, individuals manifesting type D attachment (disorganized/disoriented) utilize dissociative behaviors later in life (Schore, 1994, 2001a, 2001b).

This dorsal vagal hypometabolic energy conservation and withdrawal becomes a default regulatory strategy that occurs in helpless and hopeless situations in which the child, and later the adult, becomes inhibited and strives to avoid attention in order to become "unseen" (Schore, 2003a). In these traumatic states, which may be long lasting, both sympathetic energy-expanding and parasympathetic energy-conserving components of the infant's developing nervous system are alternately hyperactivated.

Trauma and Corticosteroids

In this dysregulated state, neural circuits in the process of development are exposed to neurotoxic levels of glutamate and cortisol for extended periods. Schore (2003a) notes that the interaction between corticosteroids (CRF, cortisol) and excitatory neurotransmitters (glutamate) is thought to mediate cell death at neurally vulnerable times such as these. Recall that, in the context of an adaptive regulatory attachment, these face-to-face emotional communications, the visual input of the mother's face and eyes, her vocal prosody, and play induce the production of *neurotrophins*, the family of proteins that induce the survival, development, and growth of neurons.

Therefore, the synaptogenesis (neural growth) and development of both the energy-expanding and, later, developing energy-conserving parasympathetic circuit is impaired. This impacts the ability to adaptively negotiate energy-expanding functions such as curiosity, environmental exploration, learning, sexual gratification, and attachment. With respect to energy-conserving functions, the ability to adaptively engage the ventral vagal system for attachment and autoregulation is unavailable to the infant and severely limited in the youngster, adolescent, and adult.

Neural Growth and Pruning

A large body of evidence supports the principle that cortical and subcortical networks are generated by a genetically programmed *initial overabundant* production of synaptic connections, which is then followed, toward the middle of the second year, by an environmentally driven process of mechanisms to select those connections that are most effectively entrained to environmental information. This parcellation, the activity-dependent fine-tuning of connections and *pruning* of surplus circuitry, is a central mechanism of the self-organization of the developing brain (Chechik, Meilijson, & Ruppin, 1999; Schore, 1994).

This process is energy dependent and can be altered, especially during the orbitofrontal's critical period of growth. Schore (1994) argues that excessive pruning of cortical–subcortical limbic–autonomic circuits occurs in early histories of trauma and neglect and that this severe growth impairment represents the mechanism of the genesis of a developmental structural defect. Therefore, this severe, experientially driven pruning of these internal limbic connections would allow for amygdaloid-driven *fear-flight states*, which would be expressed without cortical engagement of ventral vagal-mediated inhibition.

So, relational trauma in this critical period (the first 3 years of life) promotes excessive sympathetic arousal, which is reflected in excessive levels of the major stress hormone CRF, which in turn regulates catecholamine activity in the sympathetic nervous system (Schore, 1994). In reaction, norepinephrine and epinephrine levels are rapidly elevated, triggering a hypermetabolic state within the brain. In such a kindled state, excessive pruning of neurons is provoked (Schore, 2001b). The sympathetic reticular activation system is now in full flame. Unable to sustain this hypermetabolic sympathetic state, the child's underdeveloped orbitofrontal cortex reacts by engaging the dorsal vagal complex. This hypometabolic, parasympathetic state of conservation/withdrawal initiates the process of pathological dissociation (Schore, 2003a). In this passive state, levels of pain-numbing and blunting endogenous opiates are elevated, instantly triggering pain-reducing analgesia and immobility. Schore argues,

> In the developing brain, *states* [emphasis added] organize neural systems, resulting in enduring *traits* [emphasis added]. That is, traumatic states, in infancy, trigger psychobiological alterations that effect state-dependent affect, cognition and behavior. But since they are occurring in the critical period of growth of the emotion-regulating limbic system, they negatively impact the experience-dependent maturation of the structural systems that regulate affect, thereby inducing characterological styles of coping that act as *traits* for regulating stress. (p. 189)

The result is a developmentally impaired, inadequate orbitofrontal regulatory system that cannot connect to and engage the ventral vagal complex, thereby allowing for limbic-driven states, such as fear/flight/freeze, to be later expressed without cortical inhibition. This intense sympathetic state would then quickly shift into more parasympathetic activation, as the dorsal vagus attempts to shut things down. Schore (2001b) notes that "this is like riding the gas and the brake at the same time" and that this simultaneous activation of the excitation and higher inhibition results in the "freeze response" (p. 231). As these mechanisms become entrenched and stable (as states become traits), pathological dissociation in all its permutations becomes the organizing mechanism of the person's psychic functioning. Action systems, rather than being engaged with subtlety and flexibility, are engaged in the extreme.

Manifestations of Secondary Dissociation

So, how might the neurobiological impairments, noted above, manifest? Traumatized children and adults who were traumatized in childhood tend to, under stress, try to make themselves "disappear" (Schore, 2003a; van der Kolk, 1996b). Manifesting depersonalization, they experience events as if watching what is going on from a distance, while having a sense that what is occurring is not really happening to them, but to someone else. Van der Kolk notes that these *out-of-body* experiences occur when people develop dissociative splits between the "observing self" and the "experiencing self." Hence, as was begun in childhood, dissociation allows for the observation of a traumatic event as a spectator, thereby limiting or totally removing the awareness or impact of the stress or pain.

Fragmentation of Action Systems

As we noted above, dissociation, manifested in pathologically dissociated self states, enables people to develop areas of competence in certain aspects of their lives, such as work, while "dissociated aspects of the self contain the memories related to the trauma, usually leaving devastating traces in the capacity to negotiate issues related to intimacy and aggression" (van der Kolk, 1996b, p. 192). In this example, aspects of the seeking system maintain adaptive function, whereas aspects of the panic system evidence marked dysfunction. In other examples, professional competency and interpersonal sensitivity (combined seeking and panic systems) exist side by side with self-hatred, lack of self-care, and interpersonal cruelty.

Often, those traumatized by their own families experience difficulty being aware of and caring for their own needs, while being remarkably sensitive and responsive to the needs of others. Van der Kolk (1996b) notes that "unfortunately, such exquisite interpersonal sensitivity often lacks a feeling of personal satisfaction, as it is a mere replication of a survival skill acquired in childhood, and not accompanied by a sense of trust, belonging and intimacy" (p. 199).

Many repeat traumatic familial patterns in their interpersonal relationships, wherein they alternate within the roles of victim (immobilized by helplessness-triggered dorsal vagal freeze) or perpetrator (mobilized by dysfunctional rage), often justifying their behavior by their feelings of helplessness (fear system) and betrayal (rage system).

Judith Herman (Herman, Perry, & van der Kolk, 1989) notes that severely traumatized children in their adult lives tend to alternate between clinging and dependency and social isolation. Many retreat into isolation after years of frantically searching for "rescuers." Having histories of helplessness, they tend to view relationships in terms of dominance and submission. These pathological manifestations of panic, fear and rage often manifest as follows: When in positions of power, they often inspire fear and loathing; when in subordinate positions, they feel helpless, behave submissively, do not stand up for themselves, and tend to engage in alternating idealization or devaluation, at the expense of their own competence. In children and adults, the approach-mediated seeking system can also be impaired. Hence, the generation and sustaining of curiosity, learning, and intellectual pursuits may be impacted.

Studies of traumatized children have established that after exposure to trauma, children tend either to be excessively shy and withdrawn or to bully and frighten other children (Terr, 1988; Pynoos & Nader, 1988). Their inability to regulate their arousal, express themselves verbally, or attend to appropriate stimuli, combined with the pervasiveness of their emotional triggering, inhibits their ability to be attuned to their environment. Van der Kolk (1996b) notes that when trauma and dissociation compromise the ability to socialize within play, the capacity to integrate *positive* and *negative* experience is aborted. "Good and bad, power and helplessness, affection and anger continue to be experienced as separate ego states" (p. 198). Thus, dissociation fosters defensive *splitting*, precluding the ability to perceive the *gray* of life. Self and object representations are rigidly perceived as all good or all bad. In an inner world devoid of gray representations, self-blame, hypervigilance, and lack of trust prevail. These are the manifestations of traumatic, dissociatively impaired, information processing and its inherent *prediction* regarding ourselves, those around us, and our environment. Hence, these impaired information processing predictions constitute the negative cognitions, one of the cornerstones of EMDR treatment. We will return to this.

Kindling and Seizures

As we noted above, studies indicate that emotional, physical, or sexual abuse in children can lead to the overactivation of an undeveloped limbic system, ushering in a possible vulnerability to ictal (seizurelike) symptoms. Recollect that excessive pruning of cortical–subcortical limbic–autonomic circuits occurs in early histories of trauma and neglect and that this severe growth impairment represents the mechanism of the genesis of a developmental structural defect. This severe, experientially driven pruning of these internal limbic connections allows for amygdaloid-driven states, such as fear-flight states, which are expressed, at times ictally without cortical engagement of vagally mediated inhibition.

Elevated levels of CRF, resulting from childhood trauma and abuse, have been shown to initiate seizure activity in the developing brain (Hollrigel, Chen, Baram, & Soltesz, 1998; Sirven & Glaser, 1998; Wang, Dow, & Fraser, 2001), manifesting as limbic circuit hyperactivity, expressed as psychogenic nonepileptic seizures (Schore, 2003a) or partial seizures (Teicher, Glod, Surrey, & Swett, 1993).

Teicher, Glod, et al. (1993) utilized the Limbic System Checklist-33 to measure ictal temporal lobe epilepsy-like symptoms in 253 adults. Reports of child sexual abuse were associated with a 49% increase in scores, 11% higher than the associated increase of self-reported physical abuse. Reports of both physical and sexual abuse were associated with a 113% increase. Male and female victims were similarly affected.

Patterns and Conclusions in Secondary Dissociation

Frewen and Lanius (2006) posit that the results of neural activation and functional connectivity studies at a neurobiological level of analysis support the validity of the categorical distinction between primary and secondary dissociation. They note further that these differences support state/phase models of animal defensive reactions (impairments in evolutionarily based action systems) to external threat, such as fight, flight, and freeze. In other words, secondary dissociation often engages, by default, freeze, rather than fight or flight reactions. In addition, functional connectivity studies appear to indicate that although the thalamus remains online, in contrast to primary dissociation, its connectivity with cortical structures appears disturbed, again suggesting impaired thalamocortical–temporal binding (Lanius, Williamson, Bluhm, et al., 2005).

With respect to secondary dissociation, Frewen and Lanius (2006) concur with van der Hart, et al. (2006) viewing freeze as, initially, a hypervigilant and hyperaroused state of readiness. However, when stress increases or an attack becomes imminent as the sympathetic arousal becomes endangering, freeze is then combined with analgesia. Consequently, the nature of the freeze response changes to parasympathetic, becoming a dorsal vagus-mediated tonic immobility. This defensive reaction is believed to potentially reduce the likelihood of continued attack. If the continued anxiety, stress, or attack is not reduced, the analgesia and anesthesia minimize the subjective impact.

Therefore, during secondary dissociation, it seems as though at least temporarily, the mind has given up on the body and the capacity to alter the situation. Secondary dissociation becomes, by default, the solution to helplessness, manifested as a catatonoid (catatoniclike) psychological distancing of the *mind* from the *body* and of the *self* from the external *environment*.

Put another way, by default, fuguelike immobilizing trance states become quickly activated during heightened anxiety, rather than fight or flight, often leading to situations of continued victimization. Bessel van der Kolk (2006) notes that "trauma can be conceptualized as stemming from a failure of the natural physiological activation and hormonal secretions to organize an effective response to threat . . . . rather than producing a successful *fight or flight* [emphasis added] response the organism becomes *immobilized* [emphasis added]" (pp. 282–283).

Henry Krystal (1988), in a moving text on trauma, observes,

> The switch from anxiety to the catatonoid state is the subjective evaluation of the impending danger as one that cannot be avoided or modified. With the perception of fatal helplessness in the face of destructive danger, one surrenders to it . . . . in the state of surrender and catatonoid reaction, all pain is stilled and a soothing numbness ensues. (pp. 114–117)

The Neurobiology of Tertiary Dissociation

Van der Kolk, van der Hart, and Marmar (1996) define tertiary dissociation as the development of "ego states that contain traumatic experience, or complex identities with distinctive cognitive, affective and behavioral patterns" (p. 308). They also argue that ego states or identities may represent different emotions (pain, fear, or anger) or different components of one or more traumatic experiences and are therefore central to the diagnostic profile of DID.

As we noted above, if one subscribes to the position that the multiplicity of the self results solely from pathology, then the creation of self states, ego states, ANPs, and EPs is viewed as the manifestation of structural dissociation. On the other hand, if one subscribes to the position that the multiplicity of the self is normative and manifested on a dynamic continuum, from adaptive to pathological, then structural dissociation is viewed as the process that impairs the adaptive functioning of self-multiplicity, thereby mediating the phenomenon of pathologically functioning ego states (EPs and ANPs), which now function as self-hijacking alters.

Pathophysiology

Schore's (1994, 2001b, 2003b) work, in the absence of specific data regarding tertiary dissociation, views the underlying neurobiology as driven by increased amounts of trauma and parental dysregulation, thereby driving the mechanisms, noted in secondary dissociation, to further and more bizarre extremes.

At this most severe of abusive family environments, the exercise of parental power is arbitrary, capricious, and absolute. Survivors often describe patterns of punishment and coercion, such as intrusive control of bodily functions, sexual abuse, forced feeding, starvation, sleep deprivation, use of enemas, and prolonged exposure to heat or cold. Others describe being imprisoned, tied up, and/or locked up in closets. Judith Herman (1992) remarks that these abusive practices are strikingly similar to those utilized in political prisons.

Autonomic Nervous System Uncoupling

At these more significant levels of trauma, the severe underdevelopment of the orbitofrontal cortex manifests in a more profound inability at coordinating the sympathetic and parasympathetic branches of the autonomic nervous system (ANS). Generally, the two branches of the ANS are reciprocally coupled, wherein the activity of one has a reciprocal effect on the other. Hence, a sympathetic increase reciprocates a parasympathetic decrease, thereby maintaining a neural equilibrium. However, as we have already seen, at moments of marked aversive stimulation, the two branches of the ANS can also be nonreciprocally coupled. As an example, extreme fear has shown sympathetic increases in heart rate and blood pressure and simultaneous indications of parasympathetic activation in other organ systems (e.g., bowel and bladder emptying; Berntson, Cacioppo, & Quigley, 1991). Recall that in traumatized or neglected children, marked sympathetic arousal can simultaneously trigger parasympathetic dorsal vagal inhibition, what Schore (2001b) has called "riding the gas and brake at the same time," leading to the "freeze" reaction (p. 231).

However, in an atmosphere of familial terror, described by Herman (1992) as totalitarian control; violence; death threats; and the destruction of all competing relationships through isolation, secrecy, and betrayal, the hyperalternating activations of both branches of the ANS, or the simultaneous activation of both branches, at this ever-more-exaggerated level, can cause these systems to undergo an increasing *separation* and *uncoupling* (Henry, et al., 1992, Schore, 1994). This neural disconnection heralds an *uncoupled nonreciprocal* mode of autonomic function, in which responses in one branch of the ANS could occur in the *absence* of change in the other (Berntson et al., 1991). Ostensibly, the branches of the ANS become functionally *dissociated* from each other.

Self-Fragmentation and Alter Personalities

In such a neurobiological environment lacking coupled constraint, chaos is released. The resultant rapid uncoupling of the sympathetic and parasympathetic orbitofrontal circuits, if occurring continually, eventually occurs even in response to low levels of stress and is expressed in extreme emotional lability and rapid and unstable self-state *shifts*. Putnam (1988) describes these pathologically dissociative *switches* between self states as occurring rapidly and chaotically, manifesting in "inexplicable shifts in affect"; changes in facial appearance, mannerisms and speech; and discontinuities in trains of thought.

It is in this profoundly dysregulated environment that increased fragmentation of self states proliferates, creating separate *alters* consisting of complex identities with distinct cognitive, affective, and behavioral patterns. These alters tend to exhibit this profound neural uncoupling, manifested by little or no coconsciousness of each other. Action systems that have also become uncoupled are expressed in a nonintegrated and chaotic manner. The examples given for manifestations of secondary dissociation are enacted in exceedingly more chaotic and non-coconscious ways.

In childhood, numerous alters undertake specific defensive action system functions. In some cases, they endeavor to become as inconspicuous as possible by remaining still and frozen. Herman (1992) observes that "while in a constant state of autonomic hyperarousal, they must also be quiet and immobile, avoiding any physical display of their inner agitation. The result is the peculiar, *seething* [emphasis added] state of 'frozen watchfulness'" (p. 100).

In these hellish environments, these children must find a way to form attachments to their caregivers who are alternately dangerous and neglectful. They must find a way to develop some basic trust in caretakers who are untrustworthy and unsafe. They must, somehow, develop a capacity for bodily self-regulation in an environment in which their body is at the disposal of others' needs and a capacity for self-soothing in an environment without solace.

Although perceiving themselves to be abandoned to a power without mercy, they must find a way to preserve hope and meaning. The alternative is utter hopelessness, something that no child can bear. In order to preserve some faith in their caretakers, they must first and foremost reject the reality that something is terribly wrong with them. Accordingly, certain alters will go to any lengths to construct an explanation of their fate that absolves their parents of all responsibility and blame. Inevitably, then, these children must conclude that *their* innate badness is the cause. Ironically, this distortion can bring hope. In a world where one has no control, one's "badness" might be controllable. If one tries hard enough, forgiveness and change may be possible (Herman, 1992).

Emotional Action System Distortion

Thus, all action systems are profoundly impaired to the point of utter distortion. Attachments, mediated by the panic system, become bizarre, driven by young alters in the midst of severe hyper- or hypoarousal, as the fear system tries to adapt in a labile manner to severely labile conditions. Information processing malfunctions as distortions about the "goodness or badness" of one's self and one's caretakers must be created for survival. Thus, all of the abused child's psychological adaptations are geared toward the fundamental purpose of preserving his or her primary attachment to his or her parents. To that end, the abuse is either walled off from consciousness and memory, so that it did not really happen, or minimized, rationalized, or excused, so that whatever did happen *was not really abuse*. Seeking becomes necessarily impaired by perceptual constriction or distraction. Curiosity regarding the environment and the need to learn become at times oxymoronic and absurd, when in *hell*.

In adulthood, the panic system's attachment functions are often carried out in chaotic, disordered, and disorganized ways, as switching can be uncontrolled. At any time, young alters alternating with critical, abusive, or terrified alters hijack the adult self. Many adultlike but dysfunctional alters (multiple ANPs) also hijack adult function. Attachment patterns progress from disorganized to chaotic. Some alters cling for attachment, whereas others freeze at a touch. Some are frightened by sexual contact, whereas others may look for it obsessively, at times in the most destructive and shame-provoking ways.

Fear and rage systems manifest in bizarre and fragmented ways, hijacking the person into social situations that bear striking similarities to their original traumas. Those engaged in these behavioral reenactments are rarely consciously aware that they are repeating earlier life experiences. In these alter-driven, behavioral reenactments, the roles of victim, perpetrator, or both can manifest. In this climate of personality disintegration, the seeking system can also be impaired. Hence, the generation and sustaining of curiosity, learning, and intellectual pursuits are impacted.

In all this chaotic lability of emotion, identity, and function, anesthesia and amnesia are the glue that attempts to maintain order in this most bizarrely disordered state of human functioning.

Research

Although none of the research on tertiary dissociation (DIDs) specifically examined the neural circuitry that mediates temporal binding, a number of details should be borne in mind. In every disorder of consciousness that we have thus far examined (general anesthesia, coma, vegetative states, primary and secondary traumatic dissociation), the empirical evidence has suggested impairments to the thalamocortical circuitry. Consequently, it would be far-fetched to imagine that this level of neural uncoupling is not the result of severely impaired temporal binding. Nonetheless, we must await the data. The reader is referred to Reinders, Nijenhuis, Paans, et al. (2003) and Reinders, Nijenhuis, Quak, et al. (2006), two fascinating studies of tertiary dissociation that illustrate the uncoupling of the two branches of the ANS.

Society and Trauma

As we noted above, a great deal of confusion exists in both our society and our profession regarding trauma, the extent and pervasiveness of familial neglect, and the nature of dissociative processes. For centuries, society has recoiled from the notion that trauma and neglect are pervasive and found in all echelons of its ranks. Rather than understanding that our history as a human race is pervasively traumatic, we choose to believe that we have survived and adapted. We apply the same lack of vision to our children, believing that come what may, they are resilient.

Within our various professions, academicians at the most prestigious universities tell us that traumatic and dissociative disorders are the creations of therapists and false memory syndromes. Dissociative identity disorders are claimed to be *iatrogenic* (generated in the treatment situation), wherein highly suggestible patients, usually struggling with BPDs, are influenced by implicit or explicit cues or demand characteristics from naive therapists who believe in DID and have simplistic notions about memory and pathology (Loewenstein, 2007).

Frank Putnam (1995a, 1995b) has argued that the study of dissociation, and DID in particular, appears to have been held to a different standard than any other disorder. Nowhere else has such a body of research, consisting of clinical case histories; series studies with structured interview data; and studies of memory, prevalence, neurobiology, and neuroimaging, from samples of children and adolescents, from North America, Europe, Latin America, Turkey, and Asia, been so entirely discounted (cf. Loewenstein, 2007).

Richard Loewenstein (2007) argues incisively,

> When viewed through a larger sociopolitical perspective, dissociation theory intersects with many of the most controversial social issues of modern times. The role of trauma in our culture, particularly intergenerational violence and sexual abuse, crosses into historically taboo subjects such as rape, incest, child abuse, and domestic violence, and their actual prevalence in our society. In addition, the study of trauma leads us into larger legal, social, and cultural questions related to peace and war, the meaning of violence in our society, the meaning of good and evil, and even varying religious views about the relationship between men, women, and children and the nature of the family. (p. 290)

Van der Kolk, Weisaeth, and van der Hart (1996) contend,

> A hundred years of research have shown that patients often cannot remember, and instead reenact their dramas in interpersonal misery. The professionals attending to these patients have had similar problems with remembering the past, and thrice in this century have drawn a blank over the hard-earned lessons. It is not likely that these amnesias and dissociations will be things of the past; they are likely to continue as long as we physicians and psychologists are faced with *human breakdown in the face of overwhelming stress* [emphasis added], which flies in the face of our inherent hubris of imagining ourselves as masters of our own fate, and as long as we need to hide from the intolerable reality of *'man's inhumanity to man'* [emphasis added]. (p. 67)

We in the traumatology community try to shed light on this darkness, but psychological and phenomenological explanations are insufficient as long as society and science insist on functioning like dissociated ANPs. It is only through a thorough neurobiological understanding and articulation that our ideas will be given the utmost credibility. There are many in this field who believe that the nature of the attachment between child and caregiver has very little bearing on their developmental outcome and functioning. We must be able to show clearly that the unusual and often bizarre symptoms that we label dissociative disorders are the outcomes of dysregulated, *evolutionarily based, physiological action systems* that are completely predicated by the nature of the attachment between infants and their caretakers.

CHAPTER 8

Trauma and Medically Unexplained Symptoms

MYSTERIOUS MEDICAL ILLNESSES

Medically unexplained symptoms (MUS) are generally defined in the mainstream medical literature as numerous and varied somatic complaints for which conventional biomedical explanations cannot be provided by examination or further investigation. This definition addresses a lack of knowledge and seems neutral in tone. Less neutral, more strident definitions characterize MUS as physical symptoms having *little or no basis* in underlying organic disease, manifestations of emotional disorders. Recent articles in medical journals continue to recommend psychotherapy and psychopharmacological treatment, with a focus on functional improvement rather than symptom reduction.

These symptoms have been described and categorized into a group of syndromes, which include fibromyalgia, rheumatoid arthritis (RA), reflex sympathetic dystrophy (RSD), Hashimoto's thyroiditis, Graves' disease, systemic lupus erythematosus (SLE), Sjögren's syndrome, Crohn's disease, type 1 diabetes, multiple sclerosis (MS), and chronic fatigue syndrome (CFS). The list continues to grow, yearly.

Fortunately, as we shall see, these diseases appear to be explainable. As in other issues that we have already explored, the full details of the problem may not be evident, but the contours are apparent and inferable. The central character in this mystery appears to be the steroid *cortisol*, whose relationship to trauma and these diseases has been puzzling and bewildering, owing mainly to faulty empirical methodologies in its collection, extraction, measurement, and analysis. In order to understand these seemingly enigmatic medical conditions, we need to appreciate the relationships between the autonomic, endocrine, and immune systems, specifically focusing on cortisol's role in their interrelated functioning.

The Autonomic Nervous System

Recall that, in contrast to the central nervous system, comprised of the brain and spinal cord, the autonomic nervous system (ANS) is the part of the peripheral nervous system that acts as a control structure, functioning largely below the level of consciousness and controlling visceral (organ) functions. The ANS affects heart rate, digestion, respiration rate, salivation, perspiration, diameter of the pupils, micturition (urination), and sexual arousal. Whereas most of its actions are involuntary, some, such as breathing, work in tandem with the conscious mind.

Divisions of the ANS

Recollect also that the ANS is traditionally divided into two subsystems, the parasympathetic nervous system and sympathetic nervous system. The sympathetic division is energy expanding and arousal mediating. The parasympathetic division is energy conserving, homeostatic, and calm mediating. The sympathetic and parasympathetic divisions typically function in opposition to each other, though this opposition is better conceptualized as complementary in nature rather than antagonistic. As an analogy, one may think of the sympathetic division as the *accelerator* and the parasympathetic division as the *brake*. Hence, we can view the sympathetic branch as mediating "approach, seek, fight, or flight" and the parasympathetic branch as "rest and digest" and/or freeze (Dodd & Role, 1991).

Neural signaling within the two branches is mediated by neurotransmission. The sympathetic branch is catecholamine mediated, utilizing, predominantly, norepinephrine/noradrenaline, epinephrine/adrenaline, and dopamine. The parasympathetic branch is generally cholinergically mediated, utilizing acetylcholine transmission.

The Endocrine System

The endocrine system is a system of *glands*, each of which secretes a type of hormone as a chemical messenger directly into the bloodstream to regulate the body. The *endocrine* system contrasts with the *exocrine* system, which secretes its chemical messengers utilizing *ducts*, and the ANS, which utilizes *neurotransmitters* as chemical messengers. Its name derives from the Greek words *endo* (inside, within) and *crinis* (secretion). The endocrine system is an information signaling system, like the nervous system, yet its effects and mechanism are classifiably different. The endocrine system's effects are slow to initiate and prolonged in their response, lasting for hours to weeks. The nervous system sends information very quickly, generally over short distances, and responses are generally short lived. *Hormones* are the chemical messengers released from endocrine tissue into the bloodstream where they travel, often long distances, to target tissue and generate a response. Hormones regulate various human functions, including metabolism, growth and development, tissue function, and mood (Kupfermann, 1991a).

The Integration of ANS and Endocrine Systems

The ANS and endocrine system join to form metabolic pathways or *axes*. Sympathetic mediation is carried out by the functioning of the sympathoadreno-medullary (SAM) axis, wherein the adrenal medulla (on the kidneys) generates the production of the hormone epinephrine and, in combination with brainstem areas (locus caeruleus), the production of norepinephrine. When mediated by the adrenal medulla, norepinephrine is secreted as a hormone. When mediated by the locus caeruleus, it is produced as a neurotransmitter. Recall from Chapter 3 that hormones and neurotransmitters function as chemical messengers. Hence, the SAM axis is considered to be neuroendocrine, consisting of neural and endocrine tissue (Kupfermann, 1991a).

In contrast, parasympathetic function is mediated predominantly through endocrine function. The glandular mediation of the endocrine system is, generally, carried out by the hypothalamus, pituitary, and adrenal glands. These glands signal each other sequentially and are therefore considered to form and function as an axis, the hypothalamic–pituitary–adrenal (HPA) axis (Kupfermann, 1991a).

The HPA Axis and Cortisol

The HPA axis can be activated for various reasons but predominantly by the sleep/wake cycle, during stress, and for immune function. This axis functions as a complex set of direct, sequential influences and feedback interactions among the hypothalamus, the pituitary (a pea-shaped structure located below the hypothalamus), and the adrenal (or suprarenal) glands (small, conical organs on top of the kidneys).

So, for example, when the HPA axis is activated, the hypothalamus mediates the secretion of corticotropin-releasing factor (CRF)/corticotropin-releasing hormone (CRH), which then signals the anterior pituitary to secrete adrenocorticotropic hormone (ACTH), in turn signaling the adrenal cortex to secrete cortisol. When the appropriate level of cortisol is reached, its presence initiates a negative feedback on the hypothalamus and pituitary, mediating the inhibition of further CRF/CRH and ACTH production, thereby curtailing further cortisol production (Engelmann, Landgraf, & Wotjak, 2004). We will return to this.

The Immune System

The immune system is a network of cells, tissues, and organs that work together to defend the body against attacks by "foreign" invaders. These invaders are primarily microbes, tiny organisms such as bacteria, parasites, fungi, and viruses that can cause infections. The human body provides an ideal environment for many microbes. It is the immune system's function to keep them out or, failing that, to seek out and destroy them. In addition, the immune system functions to prevent cell mutations, collectively referred to as tumors or cancers.

The immune system is amazingly complex. It can recognize and remember millions of different enemies, and it can produce secretions (release of fluids) and cells to match up with and wipe out nearly all of these microbes. The secret to its success is an elaborate and dynamic communications network. Millions of cells organized into sets and subsets gather like clouds of bees swarming around a hive and pass information back and forth in response to an infection. Once immune cells receive the alarm, they become activated and begin to produce powerful chemicals referred to as antibodies. These substances allow the cells to regulate their own growth and behavior, to enlist other immune cells, and to direct them to infectious trouble spots. Under normal conditions, the immune system is able to launch attacks that destroy invading microbes, infected cells, and tumors, while ignoring healthy tissues and, when necessary, facilitating the protection and growth of cells (Male, Brostoff, Roth, & Roitt, 2006).

Self Versus Nonself

Normally, the key to a balanced immune system is its remarkable ability to distinguish between the body's own cells, recognized as "self," and foreign cells, recognized as "nonself." The body's immune defenses normally coexist with cells that carry distinctive self marker molecules. When immune defenders encounter foreign cells or organisms carrying markers that are identified as nonself, they quickly launch an attack. Anything that can trigger this immune response is referred to as an *antigen*. An antigen can be a microbe, such as a virus, or a part of a microbe, such as a molecule. Tissues or cells from another person (except an identical twin) also carry nonself markers and act as foreign antigens. That is why tissue transplants are, at times, rejected.

In some cases, the immune system responds to a seemingly harmless foreign substance, such as ragweed pollen. The result is an allergy, and this kind of antigen is referred to as an allergen. In certain pathological situations, the immune system can mistake self for nonself and launch an attack against the body's own cells or tissues, resulting in *inflammatory autoimmune* disorders. We will return to this in detail, below.

Autoimmune Structure

Lymphocytes

The organs of the immune system are positioned throughout the body. They are called lymphoid organs because they are home to *lymphocytes*, small white blood cells that are the key players in the immune system. Bone marrow, the soft tissue in the hollow center of bones, is the ultimate source of all blood cells, including lymphocytes. The thymus gland is another lymphoid organ. Lymphocytes known as T lymphocytes or T cells (*T* denotes the thymus) mature in the thymus and then migrate to other tissues. B lymphocytes, also known as B cells, become activated and mature into plasma cells, which make and release antibodies. Lymph nodes, which are located in many parts of the body, are lymphoid tissues that contain numerous specialized structures, such as T cells and B cells. Lymphocytes can travel throughout the body using the blood vessels. They can also travel through the system of *lymphatic vessels* that closely parallels the body's veins and arteries (Male et al., 2006).

B cells and T cells are the main types of lymphocytes. B cells work chiefly by secreting substances called *antibodies*, such as immunoglobulins, into the body's fluids. Antibodies ambush foreign antigens circulating in the bloodstream. They are powerless, however, to penetrate cells. The job of attacking and penetrating target cells, either cells that have been infected by viruses or cells that have been distorted by cancer, is left to T cells and other immune cells.

Immunoglobulins

Many of the B-cell-mediated antibodies created are *immunoglobulins*. Immunoglobulin G (IgG) is a type of antibody that works efficiently to coat microbes, speeding their uptake or absorption by other cells in the immune system. Immunoglobulin M (IgM) is very effective at killing bacteria. Immunoglobulin A (IgA) concentrates in body fluids, tears, saliva, and the secretions of the respiratory and digestive tracts, guarding the entrances to the body. Immunoglobulin E (IgE), whose natural job is to protect against parasitic infections, is likely responsible for the symptoms of allergy. Immunoglobulin D (IgD) remains attached to B cells and plays a key role in initiating early B cell responses.

Microphages and Natural Killer T Cells

In addition to lymphocytes, the immune system stockpiles a large arsenal of cell-devouring phagocytes/microphages and natural killer T cells (NKT cells). Some immune cells take on all intruders, whereas others are focused on highly specific targets. The immune system stores just a few of each kind of these different cells needed to recognize millions of possible enemies. When an antigen first appears, the few immune cells that can respond to it multiply into a full-scale army of cells. After their job is done, the majority of immune cells fade away, leaving a small number behind that function as sentries to watch for future attacks. In order to work effectively, immune cells need to work communicatively and systemically. At times, immune cells communicate by direct physical contact. Generally, though, they communicate through yet another class of chemical messengers, known as *cytokines* (Abbas, Lichtman, & Pillai, 2012). We revisit this in detail, below.

The Antiinflammatory–Inflammatory Balance

The immune system mediates a balance between *antiinflammatory*, neuro-protective, cell survival and growth, and *inflammatory*, neurotoxic, cell death (Allen & Rothwell, 2001; Rothwell, 1999; Szelenyi & Vizi, 2007). Therefore, an inflammatory shift in immune balance increases immune functions, whereas an antiinflammatory shift in balance decreases immune function.

The need for the inflammatory function is obvious, intended for our protection against illness and uncontrolled cell growth (tumors). On the other hand, our body also requires neural protection; at times, neural growth (synaptogenesis); and at other times, neural regeneration. We have already explored synaptogenesis in the context of our gestational and postpartum neural maturation, wherein our brain grows (in utero) and wires and rewires itself during our postpartum maturation and development. In addition, the growth requirements of our bodies necessitate the need for cell growth. We have also discovered, recently, that certain areas of the adult brain, such as the hippocampus, retain the ability to promote neural growth during learning and subsequent to psychotherapy. Indeed, neural plasticity, the central organizing force of consciousness, may very well require neural protection. Also, subsequent to injury to the body and brain, the healing process manifested by cell regeneration requires neural protection. All these functions require an antiinflammatory shift in balance. Also, during periods of acute traumatic stress, reduction in immune function is required to mediate the physiological needs of fight and/or flight neural systems. We will return to this area, below.

The HPA Axis, Cortisol, and the Immune Balance

It is at the neuroendocrine–immune interface that our central character, cortisol, emerges to facilitate the immune balance, one of cortisol's main functions (Mastorakos, Karoutsou, & Mizamtsidi, 2006). Elevations of cortisol levels suppress immune function, whereas depressions of cortisol levels enhance immune function. Therefore, when there is a need for an antiinflammatory shift, the HPA axis is activated. As a result, the hypothalamus mediates the secretion of CRF/CRH, which then signals the anterior pituitary to secrete ACTH, in turn signaling the adrenal cortex to secrete cortisol. In this situation, the negative feedback on the hypothalamus and pituitary is reduced, allowing for an increased production of cortisol, thereby *suppressing* immune function. Conversely, when a need arises for an inflammatory shift, the negative feedback on the hypothalamus and pituitary is enhanced, thereby reducing cortisol levels and *enhancing* immune function.

Cytokines and Immunochemical Messaging

The orchestration of inflammatory and antiinflammatory responses is contingent on a system of communications between the immune cells (T cells,

B cells, NKT cells, microphages) and a group of proteins, or glycoproteins, collectively referred to as *cytokines* (Allen & Rothwell, 2001; Rothwell, 1999; Szelenyi & Vizi, 2007). Cytokines belong to three families, generally referred to as *interferons, interleukins, and tumor necrosis factors* (TNFs).

Neurotoxic and neuroprotective mechanisms are closely related to the balance between the inflammatory and antiinflammatory cytokines, respectively. Hence, specific cytokines are expressed during human development, injury, and disease. Like cortisol, cytokines mediate immune function in both directions. Cytokines can be thought of as the generals of the immune army, thereby giving the orders for attack or for standing down and retreating. So, for example, when a need arises for an inflammatory shift in immune balance, cortisol levels are reduced, and inflammatory cytokine levels are enhanced, leading to the release of T cells, B cells, NKT cells, and microphages, which attack and destroy the nonself intruders. Conversely, when a need arises for an antiinflammatory shift in immune balance, cortisol levels are elevated, and antiinflammatory cytokine levels are enhanced, leading to the reduction of T cells, B cells, NKT cells, and microphages, resulting in an enhanced neuroprotective environment.

Cortisol, Immune Function, and Stress

When evolution began to tinker with our endocrine stress response thousands of years ago, stress was created by *danger*, not work, finances, the global economy, or any of our modern artifacts of stress induction. Consequently, *stress* was a situation that called for fight or flight mechanisms. From that perspective, nothing has changed our evolutionary neuroendocrine–immune response to the experience of stress.

So, if we reflect on a situation that calls for a flight or fight decision (attack, surviving a natural disaster, drowning, etc.), our neuroendocrine–immune response will be expressed as follows: (a) Our SAM axis will become activated, wherein the adrenal medulla (on the kidneys) will generate the production of epinephrine and, in combination with brainstem areas (locus caeruleus), the production of norepinephrine. These hormonal changes will facilitate an increase in blood sugars (glucose), blood pressure, and respiratory and metabolic rates. (b) Our HPA axis will become activated, wherein the hypothalamus will mediate the secretion of CRF/CRH, which will then signal the anterior pituitary to secrete ACTH, in turn signaling the adrenal cortex to secrete cortisol. The negative feedback on the hypothalamus and pituitary will be suppressed, thereby mediating enhanced cortisol production and an antiinflammatory immune balance. This hormonal change will facilitate an increase in blood volume and blood pressure, enhanced conversion of proteins and fats to glucose, and a reduction in immune function.

In situations of acute danger, these changes are adaptive, in that they mediate and fuel the usage of fight or flight options. Immune and digestive functions are reduced owing to their intensive usage of fuel and energy, changes that are adaptive in the short term. According to evolution's blueprint, danger is generally not long term; you either escape or die. However, in modern times, and in the absence of a much-needed evolutionary upgrade, our manifestations of stress can be long term. Consequently, the prolonged maintenance of the endocrine changes and persistent unneeded antiinflammatory immune balance can eventually lead to hypertension, anxiety, gastrointestinal illness, impaired healing and immune function, heart disease, diabetes, and cancers.

The Enigma of Cortisol and Posttraumatic Stress Disorder

The data from investigations of the neuroendocrinology of posttraumatic stress disorder (PTSD) have evidenced alterations that have not historically been associated with disorders of stress. Rachel Yehuda (2006) opines that the most "infamous" of these observations, lowered cortisol levels, has been the subject of much scrutiny because the finding has been counterintuitive and not uniformly reproducible.

High cortisol levels have historically been linked with stress, so much so that in the human and animal literature, the magnitude of the stress has often been defined by the level of cortisol secreted (Yehuda, 1997). Hence, high levels of cortisol secretion have been considered the de facto evidence that stress has occurred. As a result of this strong association between cortisol levels and stress and depression, it was initially hypothesized that cortisol levels would be elevated in PTSD. However, the first exploration of cortisol levels in PTSD demonstrated that the 24-hour urinary excretion of cortisol was actually lower in combat veterans with PTSD as compared to hospitalized patients with other psychiatric diagnoses such as major depression, schizoaffective disorder, bipolar disorder, and schizophrenia (Mason, Giller, Kosten, Ostroff, & Harkness, 1986). For the next few years, four of six cortisol studies verified these findings, suggesting a unique endocrine signature for PTSD.

Since then, however, several hundred peer-reviewed journal articles reporting on various aspects of HPA function in subjects with PTSD have been published, with results that have done more to confuse the issue than offer any enlightenment. These findings have indicated cortisol elevations, depressions, and nondifferences. Even in more refined methodological examinations of cortisol, spanning multiple measurements over 24 hours, the results have been mixed. Thus, when compared to controls, ambient cortisol findings for subjects with PTSD over 24 hours were found to be lowered, elevated, and insignificant (see Yehuda, 2002, 2006 for excellent reviews and discussion). Consequently, these findings have raised the question as to whether cortisol levels have any meaning. As we shall see in what follows, examining briefly the methods of collection, extraction, measurement, and analysis of cortisol will facilitate an understanding of these seemingly disparate findings.

Methodological Inconsistency

Rachel Yehuda (2006) argues that methodological details regarding how corti-sol levels were ultimately obtained are given surprisingly little attention in the PTSD literature. Although methodological issues regarding age, sex, height, weight, and menstrual status have been foci of discussion, what have been neglected are the details regarding the collection, extraction, measurement, and analysis of cortisol. The reader is referred to this article for a detailed exploration and discussion.

Yehuda (2006) notes that the fewest methodological problems are likely to result from cortisol assayed from blood samples and from measurements taken throughout the day. Yehuda maintains that cortisol levels that were measured from a single blood draw are not generally thought to provide reli-able measurements of ambient (throughout the day) levels, given that many artifacts, such as stress and varied sleep cycles, could create artificial eleva-tions of cortisol, leading to the wide range of findings. In addition, the use of repetitive venous puncture rather than an indwelling catheter (inserted once) could easily produce cortisol spikes due to even a minor unpleasantness.

Salivary samples, Yehuda (2006) notes, could have been contaminated with food particles. With urine samples, there was the additional problem of insuring completeness of collections if subjects were asked to collect samples at home. Home sampling was also problematic because it was impossible to ensure that subjects had adhered to the protocol with respect to collection times (for saliva), completeness of collection (for urine), as well as dietary or exercise restrictions. Additionally, extraction procedures, markedly more complex than with blood plasma, allowed for more error and the resultant discrepancies.

Posttraumatic Stress Disorder and Hypocortisolemia

When properly done, cortisol investigations in persons with PTSD have revealed consistent findings of *hypocortisolemia* (depressed cortisol levels). The reader is referred to Yehuda (2002 and 2006) for reviews and discus-sion of these studies. Cortisol levels in persons with PTSD were found to be reduced when compared to cortisol levels in those with depression and/or control subjects. Cortisol levels were found to be lower in subjects with PTSD as compared to controls and in combat veterans with PTSD as compared to controls and combat veterans without PTSD. Similar findings of hypocortiso-lemia were found in children who survived the 1988 earthquake in Armenia, exhibiting posttraumatic reactions 5 years after the fact. Findings of cortisol suppression were found in female adult survivors of childhood sexual abuse, as compared to controls. Finally, findings of hypocortisolemia were found in Gulf War combat veterans with intrusive posttraumatic symptoms, holocaust survivors (in excess of 50 years of the holocaust), and aging combat veterans, as compared to controls.

Subjects with PTSD and Their Offspring

Offspring of holocaust survivors (with PTSD) evidenced significantly lower cortisol excretion than offspring of holocaust survivors without PTSD symptoms. This was found to be true whether or not the offspring exhibited any PTSD symptoms. The reader is referred to Yehuda, Teicher, et al. (2007) for a listing and discussion of these studies.

In a most striking study, Yehuda, Engel, Brandt et al. (2005) reported findings of low cortisol levels in mothers who developed PTSD in response to exposure to the World Trade Center attack and collapse of September 11, 2001, and *their 1-year-old babies,* as compared to mothers who did not evidence PTSD in response to the attacks and their babies. With this study, we have our first evidence that hypocortisolemia can be caused by glucocorticoid (cortisol) programming *in utero.* Because not all children born to mothers with PTSD will necessarily develop PTSD, this finding underscores the fact that hypocortisolemia can also manifest in a population without PTSD population. We will return to the questions and possible implications of this finding, below.

What appears to be clear from the foregoing is that PTSD does have a unique endocrine signature and that this endocrine profile must have direct and profound implications on immune function. Recall that elevations of cortisol levels suppress immune function, whereas depressions of cortisol levels enhance immune function. However, in the case of PTSD, or in offspring (of PTSD sufferers), wherein the offspring do not manifest PTSD, cortisol suppression is not induced by immune needs, thereby creating the potential for an inflammatory, hyperimmune balance, in the absence of bacterial, viral, fungal, parasitic, or carcinogenic invasion.

Medically Unexplained Symptoms

As we noted above, these symptoms have been described and categorized into a group of syndromes, which include fibromyalgia, RA, RSD, Hashimoto's thyroiditis, Graves' disease, SLE, Sjögren's syndrome, Crohn's disease, type 1 diabetes, MS, and CFS.

In the absence of methodological flaws or inconsistencies, the studies of MUS consistently point at hypocortisolemia. The reader is referred to Bohmelt, Nater, Franke, Hellhammer, and Ehlert (2005) and Heim, Ehlert, and Hellhammer, (2000) for reviews and discussions of these studies. Hence, there is considerable evidence for decreased adrenal activity and reactivity manifested in decreased cortisol output in patients with a myriad of bodily disorders. These disorders have been related to stress or trauma experience, and there seems to be considerable symptom overlap among these disorders (Heim et al., 2000), suggesting a spectrum of related diseases with similar neuroendocrine correlates.

If hypocortisolemia is central to these diseases, an examination should reveal consistent findings of inflammatory cytokines and the resultant lymphocytes and antibodies in the areas affected by these illnesses. Additionally, consistent findings of inflammatory cytokines are consistent with the chronic pain that many of these diseases manifest with (for reviews, see Watkins & Maier, 2000, and Dantzer, 2005).

Sjögren's Syndrome

Sjögren's syndrome manifests as an autoimmune disorder in which the body's immune system mistakenly reacts to the tissue in glands that produce moisture, such as tear and salivary glands. It is a chronic inflammatory disease that can progress to a more complex systemic disorder that affects other tissues and organs in the body, such as joints, kidneys, and the intestinal tract.

Sjögren's syndrome is characterized by an unusual accumulation and infiltration of a particular type of antibody and/or lymphocyte in the glands that are responsible for fluid production (see Witte, 2005, for a review of such studies). Specifically, these antibodies (antifodrin and anticentromere) function as autoantibodies, given that they attack healthy tissue, not infectious invasion. Consequently, the amount and quality of saliva and tears produced decreases with Sjögren's syndrome, leading to a characteristic dry mouth and dry eyes, which are referred to as *sicca syndrome*. Other mucous membranes may also dry out. Those with this condition often have a feeling of sand or grit in their eyes, swollen salivary glands, difficulty swallowing, and a decreased sense of taste. The diagnosis is derived either from blood-work investigations of antibodies or cytokines or from biopsies investigating the presence of antibodies in glandular areas.

The disorder may present as primary Sjögren's syndrome or as secondary Sjögren's syndrome, wherein the condition coexists with other autoimmune disorders, such as SLE, polymyositis, scleroderma, or RA. Most of the complications of Sjögren's syndrome occur because of decreased tears and saliva. Consequently, people with dry eyes are at increased risk for infections around the eye and may have damage to the cornea. Dry mouth may cause an increase in dental decay, gingivitis (gum inflammation), and oral yeast infections (thrush), which may cause pain and burning. Some people have episodes of painful swelling in the salivary glands around the face. Complications in other parts of the body can occur. Pain and stiffness in the joints with mild swelling may occur in some people, even in those without RA or lupus. Rashes on the arms and legs related to inflammation in small blood vessels (vasculitis) and inflammation in the lungs, liver, and kidney may occur rarely and be difficult to diagnose. Numbness, tingling, and weakness also have been described in some people.

Hashimoto's Thyroiditis

Hashimoto's thyroiditis, also referred to as chronic lymphocytic thyroiditis, is an autoimmune disease in which the thyroid gland is gradually infiltrated by a variety of autoantibody-mediated immune processes (see McLachlan & Rappaport, 1992, and Legakis, Petroyianni, Saramantis, & Tolis, 2001, for reviews). It was the first disease to be recognized as an autoimmune disease. Hashimoto's thyroiditis very often results in symptoms of hypothyroidism. Hashimoto's thyroiditis, as an autoimmune disease, is differentiated from hypothyroidism, a symptomatic condition without autoantibody infiltration.

Physiologically, antibodies against thyroid peroxidase and/or thyroglobulin cause gradual destruction of follicles in the thyroid gland. Accordingly, the disease can be detected clinically by looking for these antibodies in the blood. Hence, Hashimoto's thyroiditis is characterized by invasion of the thyroid tissue by leukocytes, mainly T lymphocytes. Symptomatically, every organ system slows in function. Consequently, the brain slows down, making it difficult to concentrate. The gut slows down, causing constipation, and metabolism slows down, causing weight gain, fatigue, and depressive symptoms.

Graves' Disease

Graves' disease is an autoimmune system disorder that results in the overproduction of thyroid hormones (hyperthyroidism). Graves' disease is also the most common cause of severe hyperthyroidism that is accompanied by more clinical signs and symptoms and laboratory abnormalities as compared with milder forms of hyperthyroidism (Iglesias, Dévora, et al., 2009).

In Graves' disease, the immune system produces antibodies called thyroid-stimulating immunoglobulin. These antibodies bind/attach to the thyroid-stimulating hormone receptors, which are located on the cells that produce thyroid hormones in the thyroid gland (follicular cells) and chronically stimulate them, resulting in an abnormally high production of thyroid hormones (Saravanan & Dayan, 2001). This causes the clinical symptoms of hyperthyroidism and the enlargement of the thyroid gland (visible as a goiter). Approximately 25% to 30% of people with Graves' disease will also have Graves ophthalmopathy, a protrusion of one or both eyes caused by inflammation of the eye muscles by attacking autoantibodies. Other autoantibodies, thyroid growth immunoglobulins and thyrotropin-binding inhibitory immunoglobulins have, also, been observed. Still other observations have reported infiltrations of B and T lymphocytes (Wang, Chen, et al., 2007).

Graves' disease can exhibit a variety of symptoms related to hyperthyroidism, including diffuse goiter (enlarged thyroid gland), rapid pulse, weight loss, and trembling. In addition, some people with Graves' disease exhibit symptoms unique to this form of hyperthyroidism, including ophthalmopathy (bulging eyes) and, rarely, pretibial myxedema (swelling of shins). The symptoms of Graves' disease stem partly from hyperthyroidism and partly as a consequence of autoimmune self-attack.

Fibromyalgia

Derived from the Latin *fibro-* (fibrous tissues) and Greek *myo-* (muscle) and *algos-* (pain), fibromyalgia manifests as muscle and connective tissue pain and a heightened painful response to slight or moderate pressure. Other symptoms may include tingling of the skin, prolonged muscle spasms, weakness in the limbs, nerve pain, muscle twitching, and palpitations. Although fibromyalgia is classified based on the presence of chronic widespread pain, pain may also be localized in areas such as the shoulders, neck, lower back, hips, or other areas.

Other symptoms often attributed to fibromyalgia that may possibly be due to comorbid (co-occurring) disorders include the following: myofascial pain syndrome, diffuse nondermatomal paresthesias, functional bowel disturbances and irritable bowel syndrome, genitourinary symptoms and interstitial cystitis, dermatological disorders, headaches, myoclonic twitches, and symptomatic hypoglycemia. Twenty to thirty percent of patients with RA and SLE may also have fibromyalgia (Yanus, 2007).

An immunoinflammatory profile is supported by studies reporting elevated levels of proinflammatory cytokines (Maes et al., 1999; Thompson & Barkhuizen, 2003). Additional evidence for immune activation in fibromyalgia is provided by observations of increased NKT cells and T-lymphocyte autoantibodies (Fries, Hesse, Hellhammer, & Hellhammer, 2005).

Crohn's Disease

Crohn's disease presents as an inflammatory disease of the intestines that may affect any part of the gastrointestinal tract, causing a wide variety of symptoms. It primarily causes abdominal pain, diarrhea (which may be bloody if inflammation is at its worst), vomiting, or weight loss. It may also cause complications outside the gastrointestinal tract, such as rashes, arthritis, inflammation of the eyes, tiredness, and lack of concentration. Also referred to as inflammatory bowel disease, it typically manifests in the gastrointestinal tract and can be categorized by the specific tract or region affected. It can affect both the ileum (the last part of the small intestine, which connects to the large intestine) and the colon (the large intestine). Ileocolic Crohn's disease accounts for 50% of cases. Crohn ileitis, manifested in the ileum only, accounts for 30% of cases, whereas Crohn colitis, of the large intestine, accounts for the remaining 20% of cases and may be particularly difficult to distinguish from ulcerative colitis (Baumgart & Sandborn, 2007).

Crohn's disease manifests as an autoimmune disease, with inflammation stimulated by an overactive inflammatory cytokine and resultant varied T-cell and autoantibody response (Cobrin & Abreu, 2005; Elson et al., 2007). Similar observations of high levels of the cytokine TNF-alpha have been associated with the development of intestinal inflammation in Crohn's disease (Behm & Bickston, 2008).

Systemic Lupus Erythematosus

Systemic lupus erythematosus is a systemic autoimmune disease or autoimmune connective tissue disease that can affect any part of the body. As occurs in other autoimmune diseases, the immune system attacks the body's healthy cells and tissue, resulting in inflammation and tissue damage. It is a hypersensitivity reaction caused by antibody-immune complex formations. Systemic lupus erythematosus most often harms the heart, joints, skin, lungs, blood vessels, liver, kidneys, and nervous system. The course of the disease is unpredictable, with periods of illness (called *flares*) alternating with remissions (see Rahman & Isenberg, 2008, for a review).

Autoantibodies, such as antinuclear antibodies, seen in systemic lupus are directed against nuclear antigens such as nucleosomes, DNA, and histone proteins found within the body's cells and plasma. Hence, these autoantibodies are involved in the development of the disease, either by forming immune complexes that lodge in target organs, disrupting normal organ function, or by cross-reacting with targeted antigens and damaging tissue. Put another way, the systemic aspect of this disease is driven by the fact that these antibodies attack the cell, *systemically*, by attacking the nucleus and DNA. Further systemic damage is achieved by the fact that the cells of any organ system can be targeted, as opposed to specific organ systems such as those attacked in Hashimoto's thyroiditis, Graves' disease, or Crohn's disease.

Rheumatoid Arthritis

Rheumatoid arthritis is a chronic, systemic inflammatory disorder that may affect many tissues and organs but principally attacks the joints. The process produces an inflammatory response of the synovium (a lubricating fluid within the joint), secondary to hyperplasia (a marked growth in cell numbers) of synovial cells, resulting in excess synovial fluid and the development of pannus (an abnormal type of fibrovascular tissue that grows in a cancer-like fashion) in the synovium. The pathology of the disease process often leads to the destruction of cartilage and the joints. Rheumatoid arthritis can also produce diffuse inflammation in the lungs, heart, pleura (cavity surrounding the lungs), and sclera (the white area of the eye) as well as nodular lesions, most common in subcutaneous (below the skin) tissue.

Rheumatoid arthritis typically manifests with signs of inflammation, with the affected joints being swollen, warm, painful, and stiff, particularly early in the morning on waking or following prolonged inactivity. As the pathology progresses, the inflammatory activity leads to tendon tethering and erosion and destruction of the joint surface, which impairs range of movement and leads to marked deformity.

Rheumatoid factor autoantibodies (created by B cells) and T cells have been detected in the majority of patients with the established disease, as have another group of autoantibodies, including antiperinuclear factor, antikeratin, and antifilaggrin autoantibodies (De Rycke et al., 2004). These antibodies are themselves thought to be antibodies created by IgM and IgG, which have been found consistently in investigations of RA (Sherer et al., 2005). Regardless of the specifics of the autoantibodies produced, RA clearly manifests as an autoimmune disease.

Type 1 Diabetes

Type 1 diabetes mellitus (also known as Type 1 diabetes or juvenile diabetes) is a form of diabetes mellitus, appearing typically in adolescence, that results from autoimmune destruction of the insulin-producing beta cells of the pancreas. The subsequent lack of insulin leads to increased blood and urine glucose. The classical symptoms of Type 1 diabetes include polyuria (frequent urination), polydipsia (increased thirst), polyphagia (increased hunger), fatigue, and weight loss (Cooke & Plotnick, 2008). Although presenting typically in adolescence, it may present at earlier or later ages.

The process that appears to be most common is an autoimmune response (attack) toward insulin-producing beta cells involving an expansion of autoreactive T cells, autoantibody-producing B cells, and in general, the activation of the innate immune system (Bluestone, Herold, & Eisenbarth, 2010). Accordingly, examination of the pancreas reveals infiltration by T lymphocytes and B-cell-produced autoantibodies. By definition, the diagnosis of Type 1 diabetes can be made first at the appearance of clinical symptoms and/or signs. However, the finding of lymphocytes and autoantibodies is the cornerstone of a proper diagnosis. On the other hand, findings of these autoantibodies can occur prior to typical diabetic symptoms and is referred to as latent autoimmune diabetes.

Reflex Sympathetic Dystrophy—Complex Regional Pain Syndrome

Reflex sympathetic dystrophy, also called complex regional pain syndrome (CRPS), is a chronic progressive disease characterized by severe pain, swelling, and changes in the skin. Other clinical signs include edema and disturbed blood flow to the skin. These alterations of evoked pain sensitivity and swelling are not restricted to single or specific peripheral neural territories and are often disproportionate in severity to the precipitating injury. In other words, the symptoms of CRPS usually manifest near the site of an injury, which is usually minor. The most common symptoms overall are burning and electrical-like sensations, described to be like "shooting pain." People also experience muscle spasms, local swelling, abnormally increased sweating, changes in skin temperature (usually hot but sometimes cold), changes to skin color (bright red or a reddish violet), softening and thinning of bones, joint tenderness or stiffness, hair loss or hair growth, and/or restricted or painful movement.

Recently, evidence regarding increased inflammatory immune processes in the mediation of RSD/CRPS has become clearer (see Huygen, Bruijn, Klein, & Zijlstra, 2001, and Watkins & Maier, 2005, for reviews). In particular, inflammatory cytokines, such as TNF-alpha and interleukin-6, have been shown to be involved in the mediation of the pain. In some cases, these cytokines were also found externally, in affected skin blisters. Therefore, we have further evidence that although immune processes are highly adaptive when directed against pathogens or cancer cells, they can also come to be directed against the peripheral nervous system.

Most cases of RSD or CRPS originate in areas previously involved in unremarkable or noncomplex injuries, such as bruises, strains, or noncomplex fractures. In many of these injuries, minor damage is incurred by neurons, particularly to the myelin, the neural insulation around the axon. This releases neural proteins that are normally encased and hidden within the myelin sheath (Watkins & Maier, 2005). Under normal circumstances, this poses no problem. However, in an environment of hypocortisolemia and its resultant inflammatory immune balance, these harmless neuroproteins are now responded to as nonself by inflammatory cytokines, such as TNF-alpha and interleukin-6, triggering the attack of T cells, microphages, and B cell antibodies. This immune attack of peripheral nerves is consistent with the production of RSD/CRPS symptom profiles.

Multiple Sclerosis

Multiple sclerosis (MS) is an inflammatory disease in which the fatty myelin sheath insulation around the axons of brain and spinal cord neurons are damaged, leading to demyelination and scarring as well as a broad spectrum of signs and symptoms (Compton & Coles, 2008). Multiple sclerosis affects the ability of nerve cells in the brain and spinal cord to communicate with each other effectively. Recall that nerve cells communicate by sending action potentials down long fibers called axons, which are contained within an insulating substance called myelin. Multiple sclerosis can produce almost any neurological symptom or sign, including the following: changes in sensation such as loss of sensitivity or tingling, pricking or numbness, muscle weakness, muscle spasms, difficulty in moving, difficulties with coordination and balance (ataxia), problems in speech or swallowing, visual problems, fatigue, acute or chronic pain, and bladder and bowel difficulties. Cognitive impairment of varying degrees and emotional symptoms of depression or unstable mood are also common.

In MS, the body's own immune system appears to attack and damage the myelin (Compton & Coles, 2002). When myelin is lost, the axons can no longer effectively conduct signals. The name *multiple sclerosis* refers to scars (also known as plaques or lesions), particularly in the white matter of the brain and spinal cord, which is mainly composed of myelin. In MS, the inflammatory process appears to be caused by T lymphocytes. Evidence from animal models also point to a role of B cells in addition to T cells in the development of the disease (Iglesias, Bauer, Litzenberger, Schubart, & Linington, 2001). Consequently, T cells appear to react to myelin as foreign (nonself) and attack it as if it were an invading virus. This triggers inflammatory processes, stimulating other immune cells and soluble factors like cytokines and antibodies. Leaks form in the blood–brain barrier, which in turn cause a number of other damaging effects such as swelling, activation of macrophages, and more activation of cytokines and other destructive immune proteins.

Chronic Fatigue Syndrome

Chronic fatigue syndrome is the most common name used to designate a significantly debilitating medical disorder or group of disorders generally defined by persistent fatigue accompanied by other specific symptoms for a minimum of 6 months, not due to ongoing exertion, not substantially relieved by rest, and not caused by other medical conditions (Sanders & Korf, 2008). Symptoms of CFS include postexertional malaise, unrestful sleep, widespread muscle and joint pain, sore throat, headaches of a type not previously experienced, cognitive difficulties, and chronic, often severe, mental and physical exhaustion.

Antibodies, such as antinuclear autoantibodies, commonly found in other autoimmune diseases have been found in patients with CFS (see Ortega–Hernandez & Shoenfeld, 2009, for review). In addition, IgM, IgG, IgA antibodies have also been found in persons with CFS (Hokama et al., 2009).

As enhanced immune function appears to be the underlying mechanism, it is suspected that CFS may be a generalized or comorbid response to one of the immune disorders noted previously. Hence, many patients with CFS appear to have other medical problems or related diagnoses. Comorbid fibromyalgia is common, where only patients with fibromyalgia show abnormal pain responses (Bradley, McKendree–Smith, & Alarcon, 2000). Fibromyalgia occurs in a large percentage of patients with CFS between onset and the second year, and some researchers suggest fibromyalgia and CFS are related. As mentioned, many persons with CFS also experience symptoms of inflammatory bowel disease or Crohn's disease, temporomandibular joint pain, headache including migraines, and other forms of myalgia (muscle pain).

Patterns and Conclusions

We have considerable evidence for decreased adrenal activity, manifested by decreased cortisol output in patients with a myriad of bodily diseases. These ailments have been related to traumatic experience, and there seems to be considerable symptom overlap among them, suggesting a *spectrum* of related disorders with similar neuroendocrine profiles. In instances of these illness where PTSD is not present, one may suspect, given the data noted above, that these situations may suggest hypocortisolemia resulting from glucocorticoid (cortisol) programming in utero, wherein the mothers of these patients had PTSD during the period of gestation, thereby passing on their neuroendocrine profile to their babies. Nonetheless, more studies are needed to further verify this particular phenomenon.

The data from these diseases also corroborate Rachel Yehuda's explanation regarding the apparent discrepancies in PTSD cortisol studies, wherein she argues that methodological inconsistencies and flaws are the basis of the mixed results. Hence, the consistent evidence of hyperimmunity in each of these disorders is fully consistent with an underlying hypocortisolemic neuro-endocrine profile.

The data from the cortisol and MUS studies also underscore the apparent difference between somatoform symptoms of trauma (i.e., aspects of procedural memory that are expressed, or dissociated, in somatic form) and *true medical diseases* that may have trauma as a putative causative effect. As we noted above, it is crucial that we understand and are able to differentiate somatic or somatoform symptoms from these immunoinflammatory illnesses. Understanding these differences has its greatest import with respect to treatment implications. Somatic symptoms, often conceptualized as manifestations of trauma in the body, are often effectively targeted and treated with EMDR as part of a comprehensive and phased trauma treatment. However, patients presenting with psychological difficulties (whether or not trauma related) and MUS must also be referred for treatment to endocrinologists, oncologists, or immunologists, in order to attempt reregulating the hyperimmune function in these patients, which is, apparently, causative with respect to their illnesses. We revisit this in detail in the following chapter, wherein we explore the implication of these neurobiological foundations on eye movement desensitization and reprocessing treatment.

CHAPTER 9

Linking Consciousness, Neural Development, and Treatment

NEURAL DEVELOPMENT, CONSCIOUSNESS, AND EMDR

Finally, we've arrived at EMDR, as we explore the implications of the above-mentioned issues on the adaptive information processing (AIP) model and the treatment principles that emerge from it. With reflection on the foregoing material, a number of questions come to mind. How can an appreciation of the above-mentioned data and ideas help us to understand exactly how the brain and mind change during psychotherapy? How do we utilize this knowledge regarding the neurobiology of consciousness and human development to enhance our therapeutic techniques? Can this neurobiological knowledge be utilized as a central core of understanding, rather than the myriad psychological theories of psychotherapy that often are more divisive than unifying?

The answer to these questions is, thankfully, yes. As we shall see, understanding the neurobiology of the self and of human maturation and development will make clearer many of the questions that have vexed and divided our field. Is the unconscious/implicit mind important? Should the emphasis on verbal and symbolic, left-hemispheric processing that dominates our field continue? Is the relational field or vortex that surrounds therapists and patients important? Are transference and countertransference phenomena important or just artifacts of an old theory?

Exactly how the brain and mind change during psychotherapy is the fundamental mystery that the synthesis of neuroscience and psychotherapy seeks to understand. Daniel Siegel (1999) notes that, for the most part, as clinicians, we immerse ourselves in the stories and struggles of people who come to us for help in *developing beyond* old, maladaptive patterns of thought, behavior, emotion, and relating. As we have already seen, both the adaptive and maladaptive patterns that our patients bring to therapy were developed in the context of relational interactions with other selves and their nervous systems.

That is, with a few exceptions, such as cases of type I posttraumatic stress disorder (PTSD), their problems are predominantly *developmental*. Consequently, human growth within psychotherapy may very well necessitate the involvement, invocation, and strategic catalyzing of a similar developmental and relational field. Hence, this perspective of *interpersonal neurobiology*, the understanding of how our minds develop and process information in relation to the minds of others, can provide powerful insights into how the mind functions and develops within psychotherapy.

The AIP Model

The AIP model (Shapiro, 2001) is a neurobiological heuristic based on the concept of neural networks and denotes a paradigm shift from psychological toward neuroscientific theory. Hence, it serves as the theoretical foundation that explains and predicts the treatment effects of EMDR (Shapiro, 2001).

The AIP Model and Information Processing

The AIP model hypothesizes a physiologically based information processing system that assimilates new experiences into already-existing memory networks. These memory networks are viewed as the basis of perception, attitudes, and behavior. Perceptions of current situations are automatically *linked* with associated memory networks. Accordingly, AIP views information processing as the linking of neural networks related to our experience, which include thoughts/beliefs, images, emotions, and sensations.

The observations and hypotheses of AIP regarding information processing are consistent with the research findings noted above regarding neural linkage and mapping. The focus of AIP on *beliefs, images, feelings, and sensations* is consistent with neural research, in that it targets the building blocks of consciousness. In addition, the thoughts and beliefs that constitute the negative and positive cognitions, two of the cornerstones of EMDR treatment, are the *predictive* outcomes of information processing. Therefore, when negative cognitions are distorted or inaccurate, they are evidence of faulty predictive information processing. Recall that prediction, continually operative at conscious, unconscious, and reflexive levels, is pervasive throughout most if not all levels of brain function and is the predominant evolutionary product of all information processing.

Like other species of animals, we process information in order to generate predictions about the environment (safe, dangerous, poisonous, or nutritious?) and about those around us (safe, trustworthy, dangerous?). However, we humans also generate predictions about ourselves (good, bad, able, powerless?). Francine Shapiro (2001) observes that when information processing and the resultant predictions become impaired, the distortions lead consistently to *self-limiting and/or self-denigrating* predictive beliefs, generally manifested as "I'm bad," "I'm powerless," or "I'm worthless." Consequently, positive cognitions (adaptive predictions; "I'm OK," "I'm worthy," or "I'm competent") are not available in *linked form* and are therefore not believed to be true. Even when these positive cognitions are available in abstract or semantic form, their impaired neural linkage renders them isolated, thereby preventing them from being truly and *coherently believable*.

The AIP Model and Pathology

The AIP model maintains that pathology results when traumatic, stressful, or confusing events interfere with information processing and the forging of connections between diverse neural networks. The model asserts that a particularly distressing incident can become dysfunctionally stored in state-specific form, frozen in time in its own neural network, unable to connect with other memory networks that hold adaptive information.

In other words, dissociative fragmentation attributable to the effects of autonomic nervous system arousal, secondary to stress, may interfere with AIP and consequently with its associative linking of information. Consequently, when attempting to reaccess the neural networks related to a traumatic or fearful experience, a state-dependent reactivation of the same dissociative fragmentary process likely interferes all over again with the adaptive linking of the information into the present context, thereby contributing to the timeless (or frozen-in-time) nature of traumatic memories, rather than their integration into present experience (e.g., "it's no longer happening," "it's in the past," "it's over").

As a result, experiences are inadequately processed, thereby becoming susceptible to dysfunctional recall with respect to time, place, and context and to being experienced in fragmented form. As a result, new information, positive experiences, and affects are unable to functionally *connect* with the traumatic memory. This impairment is postulated to lead to a continuation of traumatic (or nontraumatic) symptoms and to the development of new triggers. As an example, a combat veteran with PTSD will likely be triggered and become fearful of an impending attack as a result of seeing a group of helicopters flying over his house. The helicopters, his past memories, and his emotional state currently and during the war are not linked *contextually* (Vietnam vs. the United States) or *temporally* (1960s vs. currently) and are therefore experienced in fragmented, unlinked, and out-of-context form.

The assertions of AIP regarding pathology are also consistent with the research noted above regarding the various forms of PTSD or structural dissociation. These data evidencing impaired thalamic activation or impaired thalamic neural connectivity, and the resultant impairment of neural linkage (spatial mapping) and neural binding (temporal mapping), are consistent with AIP's observations that associative linking of information is impaired in maladaptive information processing, thereby leading to fragmentation of memorial, cognitive, affective, or somatosensorial information.

Recollect that spatial maps are neural maps of linked information systems (oscillating at their own signature frequencies) that must be synchronized/bound with respect to frequency and temporally (in real time), thereby creating temporal neural maps. Therefore, *neural linking* is the process that brings the various fragments of information (sensory, perceptual, emotional, cognitive, memorial, and somatosensory) together, whereas *neural binding* is the process that synchronizes the varied signature frequency oscillations of the various linked fragments into a *network frequency resonance* that binds them coherently and temporally. The fact that a memory may be experienced as *frozen in time in its own neural network,* and therefore unable to connect with other memory networks that hold adaptive information, may only be a result of impaired linkage or binding, not necessarily impaired storage.

The AIP Model and EMDR Treatment

The AIP model asserts that EMDR mediates the accessing of dysfunctionally stored information, stimulating the inherent neural processing mechanisms through the standardized protocols and procedures (including the bilateral sensory stimulation), and facilitates the linking in of the adaptive information held in the other memory networks. As a result of successful treatment, it is posited that the memory is no longer isolated but properly integrated within the larger memory network. Consequently, accessing of adaptively linked information is experienced as integrated, whole, and appropriate to the present context.

From our clinical observations of the past 22 years, it is true that EMDR mediates the accessing of dysfunctionally *linked* (or bound) information, thereby facilitating the linking in of adaptive information contained in other neural networks. Thus, EMDR appears to reconfigure the neurally fragmented maps of information, allowing them to link and/or bind adaptively.

Linking PDP/Connectionism, Temporal Binding, and AIP

The models of parallel distributed processing (PDP) and temporal binding, as an overarching framework of information processing, allow us an additional way to articulate the tenets of AIP, as follows: Under optimal conditions, new experiences tend to be assimilated by an information processing system that facilitates their linkage and binding (neural mapping) with already-existing memory networks associated with similarly categorized experiences. The linkage of these memory networks tends to create a *predictive* knowledge base that includes such phenomena as beliefs, expectations, and fears. As we noted in Chapter 5, when a memory is accessed adaptively, it is linked with emotional, cognitive, somatosensory, and temporal/memorial systems that facilitate its accuracy and appropriateness with respect to time, place, and contextual situation.

Traumatic or other distressing events can be encoded maladaptively in memory, resulting in inadequate or impaired linkage or binding with memory networks containing more adaptive information. Pathology is thought to be a result of the lack of consolidation and linkage between different aspects of memory, cognition, affect, and somatosensorial experience.

As a consequence, experiences remain dysfunctionally linked within emotional, cognitive, somatosensory, and temporal/memorial systems. Memories, thereby, become susceptible to dysfunctional recall with respect to time, place, and context and may be experienced in fragmented form. Accordingly, new information, positive experiences, and affects are unable to functionally connect with the disturbing memory. Similarly, emotions, cognitions, and somatosensory sensations may also be experienced in fragmented form. This impairment in linkage or binding leads to a continuation of symptoms and to the development of new triggers.

EMDR procedures facilitate access to dysfunctionally linked experiential components, allowing them to be linked and bound and thereby integrated within appropriate emotional, cognitive, somatosensory, and temporal systems. This facilitates the effective processing of traumatic or disturbing life events and associated beliefs to an adaptive resolution.

The Eight-Phase Protocol

EMDR treatment, from the first to the last moment, whether spanning one to three 90-minute sessions or many years, is organized by a structure of eight phases. The number of sessions committed to each phase varies greatly at times, predicated by individual therapeutic needs and diagnostic situations. The reader is referred to Shapiro (2001) for details and elaborations.

Phase 1, History

A careful history is taken on a number of dimensions to identify critical targets for processing. Regarding the three-pronged approach, an exploration is undertaken to identify (a) past experiences that underlie the dysfunction, (b) present situations that act as triggers, and (c) future templates that target anxiety vis-à-vis future behaviors and functioning.

From a combined clinical and neural perspective, we utilize the history-taking to give and gather essential information. At the most basic level, we and our patients are initiating the discovery of each other, slowly and tentatively. In addition to the left-hemispheric cognitive and conscious observing that we and our patients are most aware of and comfortable with, what is also occurring is the right hemispheric-to-right hemispheric, nonverbal, non-conscious, implicit stream of expression and perception that began in infancy between ourselves and our caregivers and "continues throughout life to be the primary medium of intuitively felt affective-relational communication between people" (Orlinsky & Howard, 1986, p. 343).

With the exception of type I PTSD treatment and a few other brief treatment scenarios, this complex relational field will be the organizing core and foundation of the entire treatment, from the first moment of contact to the last session, whether we *notice* and attend to it or not. If we are to render EMDR more robust in complex cases involving personality structure, it is indeed, as Mark Dworkin (2005) argues, a *relational imperative*.

Recall that it is the *experience-driven* maturation of the orbitofrontal cortex that is responsible for the development of the temperamental dispositions that underlie our personality styles. Our biologically organized *emotional core* is biased (or conditioned) toward certain emotional responses, which are mediated by the neural templates (emotions, cognitions/beliefs, and memories) of our early attachment experiences. Hence, present life interpersonal experiences reactivate the neural maps of earlier childhood. This occurs *unconsciously* and, often, regardless of what is actually occurring, thus *biasing* or *distorting* our emotional perception of personal interactions.

Therefore, the processing of socioaffective stimuli (interpersonal, attachment, or therapy driven) is matched against earlier-formed childhood imprinted experiential neural templates, mediating an unconscious *appraisal* of the situation's emotional meaning. Consequently, perceptions of current environmental socioemotional information are computed in relation to, and biased by, the childhood-derived templates (internal unconscious working models) of our predispositional, affectively charged interactive memories and representations. We will return to this in further detail below.

In addition to the relational field that encases us, we are searching historically for the impairment in information processing that brings this patient to treatment. In many cases, specific events become apparent targets for future processing. However, in many cases, pivotal events are not apparent. Many neuroses and personality disorders develop in an environment of *ambient parental dysfunction* that may not have acute, pivotal, or keystone events. Nonetheless, the symptoms, struggles, and dynamics of these patients are always driven by impaired predictive information processing, their negative cognitions. These impaired predictive negative cognitions are one class of mislinked neural maps that must be targeted. We will return to this.

With the exception of type I PTSD, a developmental assessment is also paramount in that the fears and beliefs (predictions) generated by the developmental level that the client is functioning at will reflect targets that may or may not be explicitly articulated during the history or treatment. For example, if a client is manifesting borderline personality organization or complex type II PTSD, their predictions may very well manifest as fears of annihilation, engulfment, abandonment, and/or loss of love. These predictive fears are driven by the neural templates/maps (emotions, cognitions/beliefs, and memories) of early attachment experiences. This may not be articulated, if at all, until months or years into the treatment. The awareness of these themes by the therapist will facilitate developmentally attuned targets or interweaves and will be experienced by the client as empathic.

Phase 2, Preparation

Francine Shapiro (2001) notes that the preparation phase sets the therapeutic framework and appropriate level of expectation for our clients. Ostensibly, preparation sets the stage for all that is to follow.

In addition to the explanation of the treatment, preparation is the continued construction (begun upon initial contact) of the relational environment that will contain, maintain, and sustain our clients through their process. Regardless of their developmental needs, this environment must create an atmosphere of being heard, understood, and protected. In some cases, such as type I PTSD, preparation may be no longer than a session. In complex cases, such as neuroses, personality disorders, or complex PTSD (dissociative disorders), preparation will be *ever-present* as we weave back-and-forth between it and EMDR targeting (phases 3–6). In these complex cases, we can view it as the cycling of preparation, targeting, and repreparation. We will return to this.

Type I PTSD

The robust effect of EMDR treatment on this type of PTSD continues, after 21 years of experience with it, to be mind-boggling. In most cases, one to three 90-minute sessions are all that are needed for full symptom-free remissions. We see this clinically and through investigations utilizing psychophysiological and neuroimaging measures. Even when chronic for a decade or more, the results are the same. As an example, in working with railroad engineers (the drivers of the trains), it is not uncommon for an engineer to present for EMDR treatment after a recent fatality. It is not at all rare, here in New York, for people to stand in front of an oncoming train either by accident or with purpose. From previous experience, or from stories told by senior engineers, it is an anxious specter that is on every engineer's mind as they power up their engines for the day. Often, their working histories contain such critical incidents, spanning 10 to 15 years. We have learned that we can begin by targeting the first incident, see the immediate traumatic response, and expect it to remit in one to two 90-minute sessions. Often, we find that the recent incident was either fully or mostly reprocessed as well as a result of reprocessing the first incident, of 10 to 20 years prior.

So, why do we not see this with neuroses, personality disorders, or complex PTSD? Obviously, chronicity and the march of time are not obstacles. We have no definitive answers. However, we have enough information to make informed speculations. In type I PTSD, no matter how profound or debilitating, we are attempting to repair a neural system that had, prior to the trauma and onset of PTSD, been functioning adaptively. Therefore, the key issue here is that we are repairing a system whose premorbid functioning was intact. Hence, it needs only to be reset. In neuroses, personality disorders, or complex PTSD, we are dealing with situations that are developmental in origin. That is, they began and continued throughout the patient's neural maturation and development. Consequently, they need to be viewed as *disorders of the self*, requiring a comprehensive, developmentally oriented treatment that strives to repair or build neural structure (mapping) that was either never developed or, at best, developed incompletely. We will return to this in increasing detail throughout this chapter.

Complex Long-Term Treatment

As we have already seen, many aspects of preparation have already begun in phase 1. In addition to the description and explanation of EMDR, this phase contains processes of containment and relational management. In cases of severe complex PTSD manifesting as dissociative disorders or dissociative identity disorders, ego state work is needed to stabilize and configure the treatment to the presence of alters. To those who view the multiplicity of the self as a ubiquitous developmental line, ego state preparation may also be part of preparation for neurotic or personality disorders. So, what are the implications of the foregoing data regarding human maturation, development, and consciousness on this phase of EMDR treatment?

Unconscious Implicit Function

From the dawn of psychotherapeutic time, questions and arguments regarding the importance of unconscious and implicit function have persisted. Opinions regarding this question have divided our field and have polarized our theories and how we carry out our work. So, is there a definitive answer to this vexing question? Whether or not the preceding data are definitive, they certainly appear to be consistently indicative of the importance of nonconscious, implicit function within and without psychotherapy.

As we have seen repeatedly, our biologically organized emotional core is biased toward certain emotional responses that are, by now, driven by the neural templates (emotions, cognitions/beliefs, and memories) of our early attachment experiences (Bechara et al., 1997). Hence, present life interpersonal experiences activate the neural maps of earlier childhood. This occurs unconsciously and, often, regardless of what is actually occurring, thus biasing our emotional perception of personal interactions (Hugdahl, 1995).

Recall from Chapter 6 that emotional memory and its resultant emotions are nondeclarative, in that emotional memory is derived from experience but is expressed as a change in behavior or emotional state rather than as a recollection. Consequently, we refer to nondeclarative memory and its resultant emotion as *reflexive* and to declarative memory and its resultant recollection as *reflective*. Recollect also that Squire and Kandel (1999) have argued,

> In no small part, by virtue of the unconscious status of these forms of memory . . . arise the dispositions, habits, and preferences that are inaccessible to conscious recollection but that nevertheless are shaped by past events, influence our behavior and mental life, and are an important part of who we are. (p. 193)

We have also learned from the work of Rodolfo Llinas (1987, 2001) that the brain is predominantly a closed system whose organization is geared primarily toward the generation of intrinsic (inner-generated) images. Also, as we noted above, Marcus Raichle's work (2006, 2009) has clearly shown that the overwhelming majority of the energy utilized by the brain is for our intrinsic inner reality, whereas only a small amount is utilized to deal with any aspect of our outer reality.

We need to reexamine the emphasis that the majority of our field has placed on verbal, symbolic, left-hemispheric processing. This is not to say that we need to completely discard it but, rather, that we need to balance it with an understanding and sensitivity to the nonverbal, emotional, nonconscious aspects of perception and processing, which are invariably expressed and experienced somatically.

Recollect that, from its very evolutionary inception, mindedness (in this case emotion) is the internalization of action. Therefore, the world of *emotions* is largely one of *actions* carried out in our bodies, from facial expressions and postures to changes in our viscera and internal physiological environment. *Feelings*, on the other hand, are composite perceptions (or cortical translations) of what is happening in our body while we are in the process of emoting, along with perceptions of our state of mind during that same period.

Transference and Countertransference

If we accept the foregoing, then the phenomena of transference and countertransference cannot be ignored. To be sure, our understanding of these does need to be updated to accommodate the understanding that in all meaningful relational interactions, including the psychotherapeutic relationship, there is more going on and there is more information to be utilized therapeutically if we become exquisitely sensitive to the implicit, nonverbally expressed relational field between ourselves and our patients. We have seen clearly that maturation, development, and consciousness are mediated by an interpersonally driven neurobiology. These compelling data teach us that if we want to enhance our work with developmentally driven psychological problems, we need to see them as forms of attachment maladies, be they neurotic, personality, or dissociative disorders. Hence, applying this interpersonal neurobiology to treatment will likely require the invocation and strategic catalyzing of a similar developmental and relational vortex.

Technical Implications

The foregoing reflect broad theoretical implications to our theories of the mind and treatment. However, what does this look like in practice? How does it integrate with how we already practice EMDR?

George Engel (1988) argues,

> Interpersonal engagement . . . rests on complimentary needs, *especially the need to know and understand* and *the need to feel known and understood* [emphasis added] . . . . The need to know and understand originates in the regulatory and self-organizing capabilities of all living organisms to process information from an ever-changing environment in order to assure growth . . . self regulation and survival. In turn, the need to feel known and understood originates . . . in the life-long need to feel socially connected with other humans. (pp. 124–125)

For the most part, we know this and endeavor to be accepting and empathic. We can utilize our experiences and empathic imagination to connect with our patients. However, our knowledge of interpersonal neurobiology can help us go further in constructing a relational matrix that will enhance structural/neural growth, thereby rendering EMDR more robust in these complex long-term treatments.

Daniel Siegel (1999) notes that the capacity of an individual to *reflect* upon the mental state of another person may be an essential ingredient in emotional engagement. This "reflection on mental states is more than a conceptual ability; it permits the two individuals' minds to enter a form of resonance in which each is able to *feel felt* [emphasis added] by the other" (p. 89). This intense and intimate form of connection is manifested predominantly in nonverbal forms of communication: facial expression, visual gazing, vocal prosody, bodily movements, and the timing of responses. Siegel argues that *"feeling felt* [emphasis added] is the subjective experience of mental state attunement" (p. 149).

Projective Identification

Melanie Klein (1946) originally described projective identification as the projection of good and bad parts of the self unto an important other. This concept has evolved and received increased attention, given our recent appreciation of the relational aspects of our developmental neurobiology. The reader is referred to Bohmer (2010) for a thorough review of the evolution and application of this process.

Projective identification, through the lens of recent neurobiological findings, is currently viewed as the vehicle for mother and infant adjusting to each other's communications in a process of mutual reciprocal influence. It is, therefore, the medium of psychobiological connection and the vehicle of communication of symbiotic states that underlie the maturation and development that are mediated by the infant–caregiver relational matrix (Schore, 2003b). It is also the vehicle that our patients will utilize to communicate their nonverbal, somatosensorially expressed emotions. It is, therefore, incumbent on us to become fluent in this nonverbal somatic language.

Dissecting Projective Identification

To understand projective identification, we can break down the concept into several steps. A summary of these different steps is as follows:

1. Unmanageable emotions and feelings are experienced by our patient. These are projected into us. The aim of this process is to project these unbearable feelings, for example, feelings of worthlessness or severe anxiety, into us (or originally into the caregiver) to make them bearable or manageable. In addition, the aim and hope is for us to know and *feel* these emotions. These projections are experienced by us in somatosensorial or affective form.
2. There is an unconscious pressure on us to experience and own these feelings or sensations and to think and act in accordance with the projection.
3. If projective identification is successful, an affective resonance is created in us. Our client feels felt by us. A true affective and empathic bridge is created.
4. In this process, if we recognize the nature of these sensations and emotions and accept and notice them, we function as a container. This is then reintrojected by our client and acts as an affect-regulatory process, in the exact manner as in the adaptively symbiotic matrix of infant and caregiver (Bohmer, 2010; Ogden, 1982).

From Model to Implementation

Let us return to our questions: What does this look like in practice? How does it integrate with how we already practice EMDR?

Gabriella—Beginnings

I was beginning the preparatory phase with Gabriella, a young woman with a history of childhood abuse. Her previous treatment consisted of ego-state work (without EMDR), and she was in the process of telling me about it. Given that I intended to integrate her EMDR treatment with ego-state work, I was eager to understand what her experiences had been. As she spoke, she became increasingly anxious. After a while, I became increasingly overcome with fatigue and sleepiness. It felt like my nervous system was trying to shut down. Fortunately, in my analytic training decades ago, my supervisors stressed the importance of projective identification, particularly its use in containment and *felt understanding*. As soon as I realized that I was likely experiencing her sense of being overwhelmed and needing to shut down, to slam the brakes on her fear, my energy level began to return. That realization had, in fact, processed and *contained* the fear and need to shut down in me. I was still aware of it, in the container, so to speak, but no longer suffused by it. I continued to notice it and listen while she spoke anxiously. Not surprisingly, though, after another 15 minutes, her level of anxiety lessened markedly.

What was transacted between us was very similar to the interpersonal neurobiology that occurs in the infant–caregiver matrix. It was completely nonverbal and nonsymbolic but rather, relationally somatosensorial. It was a cry for help, soothing, and regulation, communicated in the original prototypic prosodic and somatosensory language of one right-hemispheric orbitofrontal cortex to another. What was toxic in her, her sense of being overwhelmed, was projected into me in order for me to feel it and to contain and detoxify it. At some point, approximately 15 minutes after my energy level returned, which she *felt*, she became calmer.

In a subsequent session, in the midst of ego-state exploration, Gabriella related numerous experiences of being so frightened in her childhood that she could not function. As she was becoming increasingly agitated, I said something to the effect that, "it sounds like your fear would become so great that all you wanted to do was to just shut down into a quiet emptiness." She looked at me, startled! I noticed an unusual sense of calm in me. She just looked at me *silently* for a long moment and then spontaneously remembered one of her kind teachers. Her agitation had lessened. Here, the opportunity presented itself to return her projection in a nontoxic verbal form. In both instances, she was able to experience feeling felt, which allowed her to feel understood, safe, and soothed.

Donald Winnicott (1956), in exploring this sense of therapeutic receptivity as a manifestation of the original prototypic maternal–infant dyad notes,

> I do not believe it is possible to understand the functioning of the mother at the very beginning of the infant's life without seeing that she must be able to reach this state of heightened receptivity . . . . Only if a mother is sensitized in this way I am describing can she *feel herself* [emphasis added] into the infant's place, and so meet the infant's needs. (p. 302)

This is but one example. In other cases, if we notice and pay attention, we will find ourselves feeling restless, abandoned, or unable to pay attention or focus. At other times, if we pay continual attention to our own *body scans*, other, less clear somatic sensations may manifest, initially meaningless. There will be no apparent distress visible in our patients. We may notice a subtle gasp of air or a change in our breathing. However, if we just *notice and keep noticing*, our patients' material or current interactions with us will allow our orbitofrontal to interpret them. We do not need to process this in a left-hemispheric, neurologically top-down manner to understand cognitively. We need to do what we ask our patients to do in EMDR, to just notice and let meaning transpire in a bottom-up, noncognitive manner. Even when no meaning becomes apparent consciously, our noticing and feeling will be known to our patients. Daniel Siegel (1999) notes that "our awareness of bodily state changes—such as tension in our muscles, shifts in our facial expressions, or signals from our heart or intestines—lets us know how we feel, *though bodily feedback occurs even without awareness* [emphasis added]" (p. 143). He notes further that "reflection on internal sensations may be the essential aid in knowing how another person may be feeling" (p. 272).

Mirror Neurons

So, how can these states of mind be projected and introjected? Neuroscience appears to point to *mirror neurons* as the possible mediator of this empathic neural synchronization.

Mirror neurons are a special class of brain cells that fire not only when an individual performs an action but also when the individual observes someone else perform the same action. Hence, these neurons mirror the internal state of the other, as though the observer were performing the same action. Such neurons have been directly observed in primates and other species, including birds. The reader is referred to Rizzolatti and Craighero (2004) for review and discussion.

Before the discovery of mirror neurons, scientists generally believed that our brains use logical thought processes to interpret and predict other people's actions. Now, however, many have come to believe that we understand others not by thinking but by feeling. Mirror neurons appear to let us "simulate" not just other people's actions but the intentions and emotions behind those actions. Therefore, it may very well be that nothing is being projected or introjected. Richard Chefetz argues,

> Take the changes in the experience of your body as indicating that something in your thoughts and feelings has shifted in response to something happening in your patient . . . . Be careful to remember that nothing was put into you, it was already there. (Chefetz & Bromberg, 2004, p. 429)

In humans, brain activity consistent with that of mirror neurons has been found in the premotor cortex, the supplementary motor area, the primary somatosensory cortex, and the inferior parietal cortex (Rizzolatti & Craighero,

2004). These are precisely the neural regions that would mediate internal emotional *felt states*. The neuroscientist and researcher Vilayanur Ramachandran (2000) argues that with knowledge of these neurons, we may have the basis for understanding a host of very enigmatic aspects of the human mind: "mindreading" empathy, imitation learning, and even the evolution of language. He notes further that any time we watch someone else doing something (or even starting to do something), the corresponding mirror neuron might fire in our brain, thereby allowing us to read and understand another's intentions and thus to develop a sophisticated theory of other minds.

Ostensibly, then, we are utilizing a body scan operating in the background on ourselves, making use of it as the receptive organ (apparently mirror neuron driven) of the language of the right hemisphere. This resonance of states of mind allows for the creation of a coregulating dyadic system, wherein the psychobiological state of the patient is felt by the therapist and the resulting psychobiological state of the therapist is then felt by the patient (Siegel, 1999). Thus, a matrix that mediates orienting attention, felt meaning, and optimal arousal becomes the foundation, holding environment, and container for EMDR treatment, thereby rendering it more robust with respect to coregulation and neural growth.

Phase 3, Assessment

With respect to what we have established regarding information processing, the assessment phase functions as an attempt at gathering together neural systems that are in some manner unlinked. Therefore, if we are targeting a pivotal event, we are gathering sensorial material such as pictorial memories, which are evoked when the event is recalled. We should also assess whether auditory, olfactory (smell), gustatory (taste), or any tactile memories are evoked. We assess negative cognitions, the predictive beliefs that are evoked by the memory of the event, for distortions. We look for positive cognitions as unlinked adaptive predictive beliefs and measure their believability. We then examine the feeling that is generated (anger, sadness) and measure it for subjective units of distress and for its location in the body (the actual emotion). Thus, we are gathering material from memorial, cognitive, affective, and somatosensorial systems, in order to subject these systems to EMDR sensory stimulation and processing (adaptive linkage and binding).

Dissociation and Self States

As we noted in Chapter 7, the notion of the multiplicity of the self has polarized our field with respect to its view as either normative or pathological. Daniel Siegel (1999) argues that research in child development is increasingly suggesting that the "idea of a unitary, continuous 'self' is actually an *illusion* [emphasis added] our mind attempts to create" (p. 229). So, we are still left to ourselves to decide where and when to look for the manifestation of ego states.

Those who believe that ego states are manifestations only of pathology will explore this realm only in dissociative disorders. Those who believe that ego states are ubiquitous and normative, ranging on a spectrum from adaptive to maladaptive, will utilize their exploration as a standard part of EMDR preparation. The implication of this approach is that the assessment phase should be ego-state-specific. That is, that the elements assessed in phase 3 should be targeted to a specific ego state. This alteration in technique is similar to the protocol for recent traumatic events, wherein basic EMDR technique is adapted to accommodate an inherent fragmentation of memory. Here, the inherent fragmentation of the self is accommodated.

My continued recommendation of this approach has been driven solely by the increased robustness that this approach has evidenced in working with neurotic, personality, and dissociative disorders. It is beyond the scope of this book to explore this issue further. The reader is referred to Bergmann (2008a) for a detailed review and technical elaboration.

Phase 4, Desensitization

In this phase, EMDR's sensory stimulation, in visual, auditory, or tactile form, is utilized along with various procedural elements to desensitize the disturbance of the cognitive, affective, memorial, and somatosensorial elements of the issue being targeted. The reader is referred to Shapiro (2001) for details and elaboration.

State Versus Trait Change

Recall that during maturation and development, emotional *states* that are continuously maintained eventually become characterological *traits*, constituting the scaffolding of intrapsychic and interpersonal functioning. Therefore, calm and continuously regulated states eventually become traits of self-regulation. Conversely, traumatic and chronically dysregulated states, if maintained and not reregulated, eventually become traits of dysregulation.

In EMDR, we attempt to facilitate just enough state change to eventually facilitate a consistent trait change. In type I PTSD, the sensory stimulation, predominantly, along with the procedural steps, combined with our calm and understanding demeanor, appears to suffice as the needed state change that quickly brings about the remission of symptoms and the desired trait change.

Neurotic, Personality, and Dissociative Disorders

Recall that in neuroses, personality disorders, or complex PTSD, we are dealing with situations that are developmental in origin. That is, they began and have continued throughout the patient's neural maturation and development. Consequently, they need to be viewed as disorders of the self, requiring a developmentally oriented treatment that strives to repair or build neural structure (mapping) that was either never developed or, at best, developed incompletely.

The relational elements that were explored regarding the preparation phase are equally, if not more, important here. Our ability to notice our own body scan and trust it to be the receptive instrument of nonconscious communication from our patients will keep us in a felt empathy with their nervous system and self (or selves). This resonance of states of mind will continue to maintain a coregulating dyadic system. Ostensibly, this felt relational matrix functions as a *developmentally adaptive state change* that will, more robustly, in combination with EMDR targeting (phases 3–6), facilitate a developmentally derived trait change. So, how does this look during EMDR targeting?

Gabriella—Revisited

In the midst of a session, wherein Gabriella and a young ego state were processing a belief regarding self-defect ("there's something very wrong with me"), she became extremely upset, shaking and crying inconsolably. Attempts at inner dialogue and self-soothing were only minimally effective. She cried, shook, and looked at me imploringly. I noticed a discomfort in me, initially faint but gradually increasing. I felt uncomfortable in my own skin. It was difficult to think and to sit still. I just kept noticing it, suspecting that I was resonating some aspect of her inner experience. Suddenly, I gasped, found that my breathing deepened as I exhaled, and after a minute or so, noticed that her previously shallow breathing also deepened somewhat. She continued crying, but the shaking was gradually subsiding. Not surprisingly, the sensation in me was also subsiding. I was wondering whether I should try to verbalize in some way what had just occurred. Continuing to cry, she spontaneously resumed processing. That answered my question. This was to remain felt between us but unspoken, for now.

Relational Mirroring

Again, what was overwhelming and toxic for Gabriella was conveyed to me in order to for me to know, feel, contain, and detoxify. My noticing and resultant containment of this experience was likely mirrored in her, thereby soothing her somewhat, and reregulated her. Lewis Aron (1998) notes that gradually, patient and therapist "mutually regulate each other's behaviors, enactments, and states of consciousness such that each gets under the other's skin, each reaches the other's guts, each is breathed in and absorbed by the other" (p. 26). Similarly, Sands (1997) offers that our patients are motivated to communicate these unarticulated experiences to us, through projective identification, in order to "have one's communication be viscerally received, contained, 'lived through,' symbolized, and given back in such a way that one knows the patient from the 'inside out'"(p. 26).

It is now neuroscience, in addition to psychoanalytic theory, that is impressing on us to not ignore the fact that affect recognition initially takes place on a bodily level, wherein we feel in our body's reactions something of what the other person feels and convey this recognition through our bodily responses, such as a sudden gasp or a change in our breath, posture, or facial expression. In sum, neuroscience is telling us to have our patients be more aware of what is transpiring in their bodies, that is, to notice their bodily expressed emotions as much as, if not more than, their feelings. It is telling us to do the same. Phillip Bromberg (1998c) posits incisively that "dissociated experience thus tends to remain unsymbolized by thought and language, exists as a separate reality outside of self-expression, and is cut off from . . . the rest of the personality" (p. 133).

Relational Resonance

Daniel Siegel (1999), in a compelling and lucid synthesis of subjective experience, neuroscience, and the interpersonal context of self-development, argues that engrained dysfunctional patterns of self-organization require an interpersonal relationship in psychotherapy, wherein,

> A therapist and patient enter into a resonance of states of mind, which allows for the creation of a co-regulating dyadic system . . . . In this way, there is a direct resonance between the primary emotional, psychobiological state of the patient and that of the therapist. These nonverbal expressions are mediated by the right hemisphere of one person and perceived by the right hemisphere of the other. (p. 298)

Put another way, this coregulating dyad, created by this mutual resonance, may likely be the closest replication of the original dyad. Hence, we may be creating the best facsimile of the original state of neural structuralization, which then grounds and invigorates EMDR.

In either case, the lesson for us is that if we do not find a way to work with these body-based transferences and countertransferences, this material will never enter EMDR treatment and will continue to bog it down and reduce its robustness.

Phase 5, Installation

In phase 5, the positive cognition is either reaffirmed or refined and subjected to EMDR's sensory stimulation for strengthening until the validity of cognition (VOC) reaches an ideal of 7. The reader is referred to Shapiro (2001) for detail and elaboration. The foregoing, if it manifests during installation, applies as well. In general, though, if it is dealt with in preparation and desensitization, the odds are that by the time we arrive at installation, there should little if any of it occurring.

Phase 6, Body Scan

After the positive cognition has been fully installed, the client is asked to hold in mind both the target and the positive cognition and scan his or her body from top to bottom. Any residual discomforting sensations are then targeted with sensory stimulation until cleared. The reader is referred to Shapiro (2001) for detail and elaboration.

It is here that we utilize the organ of emotional expression to insure that our work is complete. Reflecting on the foregoing also informs us that we could do more of this during the other phases as well. Ostensibly, even if the processing appears to be progressing well, occasionally asking "*what* do you notice in your body" or "*where* do you notice *that* in your body" will surely enhance the processing, without getting in the way. In addition, during the body scan, we should ask ourselves the same question and then notice and feel.

Phase 7, Closure, and Phase 8, Reevaluation

If the foregoing occurs in these phases, it is dealt with in the exact manner as noted above. The important piece to be kept in mind, for us, is to see, listen, and most important, *notice, feel, and notice some more.*

SOMATOFORM SYMPTOMS VERSUS MEDICALLY UNEXPLAINED SYMPTOMS

As was noted above, given the myriad manifestations of somatic symptoms and medical illnesses that many of our patients present with, it is crucial that we understand and are able to differentiate somatic or somatoform symptoms from the immunoinflammatory illnesses, which are now referred to as *medically unexplained symptoms* (MUS). This group of illnesses includes fibromyalgia, rheumatoid arthritis, reflex sympathetic dystrophy, Hashimoto's thyroiditis, Graves' disease, systemic lupus erythematosus, Sjögren's syndrome, Crohn's disease, type 1 diabetes, multiple sclerosis, and chronic fatigue syndrome.

Understanding these illnesses and their differentiation from other somatoform symptoms has its greatest import with respect to treatment implications. Somatic symptoms, often conceptualized as manifestations of trauma in the body, are often effectively targeted and treated with EMDR, as part of a comprehensive and phased treatment. However, patients presenting with psychological difficulties (whether or not trauma related) and MUS must also be referred for treatment to endocrinologists, oncologists, or immunologists in order to attempt to reregulate the hyperimmune function in these patients, which is apparently causative with respect to their illnesses.

Medically Unexplained Symptoms and Medical Treatment

Hashimoto's thyroiditis and Graves' disease are initially treated symptomatically. Hashimoto's thyroiditis is treated as *hypothyroidism* with thyroid hormone. Graves' disease is treated as *hyperthyroidism* with antithyroid medications or radioactive iodine.

The other illnesses are generally treated with medications that suppress immune function. One line of treatment is the use of hydrocortisone as a method of suppressing the immune system. Recall that elevations of cortisol reduce immune function.

Another line of treatment is the utilization of various antiinflammatory interferons, interleukins, and tumor necrosis factors. These cloned cytokines attempt to mimic our own antiinflammatory cytokines, which mediate the suppression of immune function.

A third line of treatment is the use of antiinflammatory antibodies, such as intravenous immunoglobulin. Recently, a new line of medications referred to as antiinflammatory monoclonal antibodies have been developed through cloning and have shown promising results.

The overall results of these treatments have been mixed. No apparent reason has been found as to why some patients respond well, moderately, or not at all. However, if we reflect on the data that were presented in Chapter 8, a number of speculative possibilities become apparent.

Recall that hypocortisolemia can be caused by glucocorticoid (cortisol) programming *in utero*. Because not all children born to mothers with PTSD will necessarily develop PTSD, this finding underscores the fact that hypocortisolemia can also manifest in a population without PTSD. It is therefore possible that patients who do respond well to the treatments noted may manifest hypocortisolemia but not PTSD. This is certainly a line of inquiry that research needs to investigate. The data do underscore that if patients with MUS do manifest a trauma history, the PTSD must be treated, in that it apparently mediates the hypocortisolemia.

Medically Unexplained Symptoms and EMDR Treatment

In addition to the treatment of underlying traumas, a number of other issues need to be kept in mind. At times, the extreme stress and discomfort of the medical treatment of these illnesses often need to be dealt with initially.

The treatment itself can be disturbing. In some cases, these medical treatments become traumas themselves, when the wrong treatment is applied.

Recall that if one searches through the data on MUS, or PTSD for that matter, without the ability to discern proper methodologies, one is likely to find studies that point to hypocortisolemia or hypercortisolemia as well as studies that indicate that cortisol has no bearing. Unfortunately, endocrinologists, oncologists, or immunologists are not always able to discern empirical methodological flaws in published studies. Regrettably, many assume that peer-reviewed articles are always properly screened for design flaws. As a result, it is not *rare* that patients with MUS will be improperly treated with *inflammatory* immunoglobulins or cytokines if physicians are being informed by data that claim that MUS are driven by hypercortisolemia. Again, this is not common, but it is hardly rare.

Conclusions

With reflection on the foregoing, a number of issues become clear. Adaptive information processing (AIP) is a robust model that reflects the major aspects of neural mapping and information processing. It is configured to target memory, predictive cognition, and the affective nature of feelings and emotions. To its credit, it also implicitly differentiates between *emotions*, which are somatically expressed, and *feelings*, the cortically expressed translations of emotions. The only minor correction that it appears to require is the reconceptualization of impaired memorial storage to impaired memorial linkage and/or binding.

The data on maturation, development, and attachment suggest strongly that we not ignore nonconscious, implicit, and relational phenomena, areas of focus that have traditionally been relegated to psychodynamic treatment. Robert Shaw (2004) argues that our field has examined the role of the body in psychotherapy, but the focus has been almost exclusively on the patient's bodily experience. As a result, the "therapist's body is largely absent, as though there is only one body in the consulting room" (p. 272). The two vignettes from Gabriella's treatment are dramatic examples of the power of the relational field, operating at an *embodied*, nonverbal level and accessed through the therapist's ongoing body scan.

Traditionally, in the absence of neurobiological data, our choices of practice paradigms have been predicated by our opinions and those of our teachers. However, our discovery and embracing of EMDR has taught us to think differently and continue to *observe* rather than follow mainstream opinions. Let us continue to learn from this experience and allow these new data to take us beyond the debates between the various competing schools of psychological thought.

CHAPTER 10

Closing Thoughts

Throughout the chapters of this book, we have examined neuroplasticity as it manifests in maturation, development, information processing, and their disorders. We have seen that the growth, development, and integration of neural networks, as manifestations of neuroplasticity, are the mechanisms underlying consciousness, parenting, interpersonal relationships, and the healing process of psychotherapy.

EVOLUTION'S GLORY

Today, neuroplasticity is increasingly understood, within limits, to be an underlying mechanism of neurofunction at any age. The adult brain appears to possess a tendency toward neural *stabilization*, while at the same time, it maintains a potential for plastic *reorganization*. More and more, we see evidence that the brain is capable of reorganization in response to changes in stimulation. Some examples of these changes are dramatic and result, in great part, from the application of sensory stimulation. The robust effect of EMDR in type I posttraumatic stress disorder is one such example. In 90 minutes, the profound disorganization of thalamic function and neural mapping is reversed by *sensory stimulation and noticing*. The reader is referred to Bergmann (2008b, 2010) for details and elaboration on EMDR's theorized impact on the repair of temporal binding.

Another example of the capability of the brain's dramatic reorganization is from cases of vestibular damage, rendering people unable to maintain balance and spatial orientation. The original successful treatment of such cases entailed a construction hard hat containing a machine, invented by Paul Bach-y-Rita, a scientist and rehabilitation physician, which sent electrical impulses to a plastic strip that was placed on the tongue. Within moments, the symptoms ceased. After 20 minutes, the results were maintained without the hat in excess of 20 additional minutes. Hence, the tongue, in combination with the neural stimulation, acted as a secondary road (neural map) to vestibular function. An entire neural circuit had been reorganized (Bach-y-Rita, 1972;

Doidge, 2007). Currently still in use, this machine has been reduced drastically in size, and is sold under the name Brainport. After a 20-minute treatment, the effects now appear to last for hours.

Paul Bach-y-Rita's first invention, in the 1960s, was a chair device that converted video images from a television camera into vibratory tactile patterns that were *displayed* as 400 points of vibration on the user's back. This allowed congenitally blind people, with retinal damage, to read, make out faces and shadows, react to and avoid objects that were thrown at them, and measure distance (Bach-y-Rita, Collins, Saunders, White, & Scadden, 1969; Doidge, 2007). The development and production of this device was typically resisted by mainstream science because contemporary neural science could not explain the *theoretical possibility* of such success. However, Bach-y-Rita continued to develop this machinery and reduce its size, as well. The plate on the back of the chair was reduced to a paper-thin strip of plastic, the diameter of a silver dollar that is placed on the tongue. The computer was reduced radically, and the camera, once the size of a suitcase, could now be strapped onto the frame of one's eyeglasses. Thirty years after his original machine, scientists using this modern version have scanned patients' brains and have confirmed that the tactile images that enter their brain via a camera and then through their tongues are indeed processed by their visual cortices (Chebat, Rainville, Kupers, & Ptito, 2007).

Thus, we see dramatic examples indicating that the brain, far from being an ensemble of specialized parts, each preset in its location and role, is in fact a dynamic organ that can rewire itself, in many cases, as the need arises. Further, the common *catalyst* in these fantastic situations appears to be sensory stimulation.

EVOLUTION'S COMPROMISE

We have also seen that our brain is the product of millions of years of evolutionary adaptation, wherein older structures and mechanisms were conserved and modified, whereas newer structures were created, developed, and expanded. Although much of this conservation and development has created a fascinating, efficient, and brilliant organ of consciousness, some aspects of evolution's compromises in design have created a fertile ground for the disturbance of these neural systems.

As we have discovered, evolution appears to be guided and driven, first and foremost, by the prime directive of the physical survival of the species. In service of this edict, compromises in our neural design appear to have been made, resulting in an overriding intrinsic functioning that is organized around primitive *reflexive* flight-or-fight mechanisms rather than a *reflective* conscious and reality-based emphasis. Interpreting the present, reflexively, on the basis of past experience is quick and adaptive in the "jungle." *Overreacting* in this context is more adaptive than *underreacting*. However, in the "village" and in the "home," the predominance of nonconscious, implicit perception and reflexive decision-making can wreak havoc on intrapsychic and interpersonal functioning.

By default, and before we experience functional or dysfunctional parenting, our immature brains are wired to look for danger and pay more attention to the unpleasant than the pleasant. For example, 1 negative criticism will override 10 compliments. This aspect of evolution's prewired plasticity combined with the effects of maturation and development render plasticity, paradoxically, to be causative in *rigidity* as well as *flexibility*.

Recall that during maturation and development, emotional *states* that are continuously maintained eventually become characterological *traits*, constituting the scaffolding (neural maps) of intrapsychic and interpersonal functioning. Therefore, calm and continuously regulated states eventually become traits (neural maps) of self-regulation. Conversely, traumatic and chronically dysregulated states, if maintained and not reregulated, eventually become traits of dysregulation. In this profoundly formative developmental environment, "once a particular plastic change occurs in the brain and becomes well established, it can prevent other changes from occurring" (Doidge, 2007, p. xx). Thus, it is the combination of evolution's preset maps (reflexive fight-flight), which are not designed to be plastic, and the profound effect of our original developmental attachment on neural structure that renders the treatment of self-disorders, to this point, so difficult and lengthy.

THE CHALLENGE FOR TREATMENT

The treatment of type I posttraumatic stress disorder with EMDR has been a continuously joyful and miraculous experience that has not diminished in the past 21 years. However, treating characterological (neurotic, personality and dissociative) maladies, although more robust since the advent of EMDR, continues to be challenging and slow. Pending discoveries that will enhance neuroplastic change, we need to find additional ways to further catalyze this process.

Louis Cozolino (2002) argues incisively that if we are to enhance neural plasticity, we need to find ways to invoke a *neural sensitivity* that is similar to the prototypic neural sensitivity of maturation and development. Consequently, in addition to our techniques, we are challenged to find ways to create a neural synchronization of our patients' and our own nervous systems.

The major implication of the enormous amount of neurobiological attachment data on therapeutic technique points toward the understanding and harnessing of projective identification as the mechanism of neural synchronization. Arizmendi (2008), citing Gallese (2003), describes this process as,

... an empathic, intersubjective communication process that is completely implicit and automatic, relying on *prereflexive* action simulation (at the neurological level) that connects the observed with the observer. In brief, neuroscientists are finding that the process of observing another's actions (e.g., body posture, facial expressions, speech, etc.) creates a simulated experiential state in the body of the observer (embodied simulation) via the work of mirror neurons. In essence, our states of empathic attunement are grounded in our body experiences and this happens automatically, without conscious effort beyond that of listening and observing. (p. 446)

Note that this takes place at a prereflexive level, taking us beyond the limitations of focusing exclusively on cognitive reflective phenomena. Ironically, this technique is not foreign or radical vis-à-vis EMDR. In essence, we are taking the body scan and applying it to ourselves throughout the session. These regulated emotional exchanges, expressed and perceived by our patients' bodies and our own bodies, are likely to trigger synchronized energy shifts, which are the prototype for structural neural growth. Therefore, the results can be far-reaching, quite possibly creating a facsimile that is as close as possible to the original dyadic matrix of neural organization, harnessing it as the *neural sensitivity state change* that will facilitate a more robust EMDR and neural reorganization.

If evolution has deemed that we function at our *core* in a reflexive manner, then it would seem imperative that EMDR treatment (or any other treatment approach) be enhanced by an adaptive reflexive medium that dovetails with our essential reflexive core. That reflexive medium appears to be the relational field that is manifested by the implicit and embodied communications that are passing back and forth between our patients and us. It may be the catalyst that enhances the neural plasticity that will render our treatment increasingly robust. Many of EMDR's treatment principles and interweaves regarding complex treatment have been derived from observations of EMDR at its most robust. Let us use the same principle and try to insert into our work the relational vortex that may somewhat replicate the original robust environment of neural plasticity and growth.

References

Abbas, A. K., Lichtman, A. H., & Pillai, S. (2012). *Cellular and molecular immunology* (7th ed.). New York, NY: Elsevier.

Albright, T. D., Jessel, T. M., Kandel, E. R., & Poser, M. I. (2001). Progress in the neural sciences in the century after Cajal (and the mysteries that remain). *Annals of the New York Academy of Sciences, 929*, 11–40.

Alkire, M. T. (2009). General anesthesia and consciousness. In S. Laureys & G. Tononi (Eds.), *The neurology of consciousness* (pp. 118–134). New York, NY: Elsevier, Academic Press.

Allen, S. M., &. Rothwell, N. J. (2001). Cytokines and acute neurodegeneration. *National Review of Neurosciences, 2*, 734–744.

Alvarez, P., & Squire, L. R. (1994) Memory consolidation and the medial temporal lobe: A simple network model. *Proceedings of the National Academy of Sciences, USA, 91*, 7041–7045.

Akshoomoff, N. A., & Courchesne, E. (1992). A new role of the cerebellum in cognitive operations. *Behavioral Neuroscience, 106*, 731–738.

Akshoomoff, N. A., & Courchesne, E. (1994). Intramodality shifting attention in children with damage to the cerebellum. *Journal of Cognitive Neuroscience, 6*, 388–399.

Anand, K. J. S., & Aynsley–Green, A. (1985). Metabolic and endocrine effects of surgical ligation of patent ductus arteriosus in the human preterm neonate: Are there implications for further improvement of postoperative outcome? *Modern Problems in Paediatrics, 23*, 143–57.

Anand, K. J. S., & Carr, D. B. (1989). The neuroanatomy, neurophysiology, and neurochemistry of pain, stress, and analgesia in newborns and children. *Pediatric Clinics of North America 36*(4), 795–822.

Anderson, J. A. (1973). The theory for the recognition of items from short memorized lists. *Psychological Review, 80*, 417–438.

Anderson, J. A. (1977). Neural models with cognitive implications. In D. LaBerge & S. J. Samuels (Eds.), *Basic processes in reading perception and comprehension* (pp. 27–90). Hillsdale, NJ: Erlbaum.

Andreasen, N. C. (1985). Posttraumatic stress disorder. In H. I. Kaplan & B. J. Saddock (Eds.), *Comprehensive textbook of psychiatry* (4th ed., pp. 918–924). Baltimore, MD: Williams & Wilkins.

Andreasen, N. C., O'Leary, D. S., Arndt, S., Cizadlo, T., Hurtig, R., Rezai, G. L., . . . Hichwa, R. D. (1995). Short-term and long-term verbal memory: A positron emission tomography study. *Proceedings of the National Academy of Sciences, 92*, 5111–5115.

Arizmendi, T. G. (2008). Nonverbal communication in the context of dissociative processes. *Psychoanalytic Psychology, 25*(3), 443–457.

Arnsten, A. F. T., Steere, J. C., & Hunt, R. D. (1996). The contribution of noradrenergic mechanisms to prefrontal cortical cognitive function: Potential significance for attention-deficit hyperactivity disorder. *Archives of General Psychiatry, 53,* 448–455.

Aron, L. (1998). The clinical body and the reflexive mind. In L. Aron & F. S. Anderson (Eds.), *Relational perspectives on the body* (pp. 3–37). Hillsdale, NJ: Analytic Press.

Awh, E., Smith, E. E., & Jonides, J. (1995). Human rehearsal process and the frontal lobes: PET evidence. *Annals of the New York Academy of Sciences, 1769,* 97–117.

Bach-y-Rita, P. (1972). *Brain mechanisms and sensory substitutions.* New York, NY: Academic Press.

Bach-y-Rita, P., Collins, C. C., Saunders, F. A., White, B., & Scadden, L. (1969). Vision substitution by tactile image projection. *Nature, 221*(5184), 963–964.

Bailey, C. H., Bartsch, D., & Kandel, E. R. (1996). Toward a molecular definition of long-term memory storage. *Proceedings of the National Academy of Sciences, 93,* 13445–13452.

Bailey, C. H., & Chen, M. (1983). Morphological basis of long-term habituation and sensitization in Aplysia. *Science, 220,* 91–93.

Basar, E., Basar–Eroglu, C., Karakas, S., & Schürmann, M. (2000). Brain oscillations in perception and memory. *International Journal of Psychophysiology, 35*(2–3), 95–124.

Basar, E., Basar–Eroglu, C., Karakas, S., & Schürmann, M. (2001). Gamma, alpha, delta, and theta oscillations govern cognitive processes. *International Journal of Psychophysiology, 39,* 241–248.

Baumgart, D. C., & Sandborn, W. J. (2007). Inflammatory bowel disease: clinical aspects and established and evolving therapies. *The Lancet, 369,* 1641–1657.

Beebe, B., & Lachmann, F. (1992). The contribution of mother–infant mutual influence to the origins of self and object representations. In N. J. Skolnick & S. C. Warshaw (Eds.), *Relational perspectives in psychoanalysis* (pp. 83–117). Hillsdale, NJ: Analytic Press.

Bechara, A., Damasio, H., Tranel, D., & Damasio, A. R. (1997). Deciding advantageously before knowing the advantageous strategy. *Science, 275,* 1293–1295.

Behm, B. W., & Bickston, S. J. (2008). Tumor necrosis factor-alpha antibody for maintenance of remission in Crohn's disease. *Cochrane Database of Systematic Reviews,* Issue 1, Art. No. CD006893.

Bell, M. L. (1997). Postoperative pain management for the cognitively impaired older adult. *Seminars in Perioperative Nursing* 6(1), 37–41.

Bennett, M. V. L. (1997). Gap junctions as electrical synaptic. *Journal of Neuropsychology, 26,* 349–366.

Bergmann, U. (2008a). Hidden selves: Treating dissociation in the spectrum of personality disorders. In C. Forgash & M. Copeley (Eds.), *Healing the heart of trauma and dissociation with EMDR and ego state therapy* (pp. 227–266). New York, NY: Springer Publishing Company.

Bergmann, U. (2008b). The neurobiology of EMDR: Exploring the thalamus and neural integration. *Journal of EMDR Practice and Research, 2*(4), 300–314.

Bergmann, U. (2010). EMDR's neurobiological mechanisms of action: A survey of 20 years of searching. *Journal of EMDR Practice and Research, 4*(1), 22–42.

Berne, E. (1957a). Ego states in psychotherapy. *American Journal of Psychotherapy, 11,* 293–390.

Berne, E. (1957b). Intuition v. the ego image. *Psychiatric Quarterly, 31,* 611–627.

Berne, E. (1961). *Transactional analysis in psychotherapy: A systematic individual and social psychiatry.* New York, NY: Grove Press.

Berntson, G. G., Cacioppo, J. T., & Quigley, K. S. (1991). Autonomic determinism: The modes of autonomic control, the doctrine of autonomic pace, and the laws of autonomic constraint. *Psychological Review, 98,* 459–487.

Besson, C., & Louilot, A. (1995). Asymmetrical involvement of mesolimbic dopaminergic neurons in affective perception. *Neuroscience, 68,* 963–968.

Bienenstock, E., & von der Malsburg, C. (1986). Statistical coding and short-term synaptic plasticity: A scheme for knowledge representation in the brain. In E. Bienenstock, F. Fogelman, & G. Weisbuch (Eds.), *Disordered systems and biological organization* (pp. 247–272). Les Houches, France: Springer–Verlag.

Blanck, G., & Blanck, R. (1974). *Ego psychology: theory and practice.* New York, NY: Columbia University Press.

Block, N. (2005). Two neural correlates of consciousness. *Trends in Cognitive Sciences, 9,* 46–52.

Bluestone, J. A., Herold, K., & Eisenbarth, G. (2010). Genetics, pathogenesis and clinical interventions in Type 1 diabetes. *Nature, 464*(7293), 1293–1300.

Bohmelt, A. H., Nater, U. M., Franke, S., Hellhammer, D. H., & Ehlert, U. (2005). Basal and stimulated hypothalamic–pituitary–adrenal axis activity in patients with functional gastrointestinal disorders and healthy controls. *Psychosomatic Medicine, 67,* 288–294.

Bohmer, M. W. (2010). Communication by impact and other forms of non-verbal communication: A review of transference, countertransference and projective identification. *African Journal of Psychiatry, 13,* 179–183.

Bradley, L. A., McKendree–Smith, N. L., & Alarcon, G. S. (2000). Pain complaints in patients with fibromyalgia versus chronic fatigue syndrome. *Current Review in Pain, 4*(2), 148–157.

Braitenberg, V. (1978). Cell assemblies in the cerebral cortex. In R. Heim & G. Palm (Eds.), *Architectonics of the cerebral cortex. Lecture notes in biomathematics 21, theoretical approaches in complex systems* (pp. 171–188). Berlin: Springer–Verlag.

Breau, L. M., Camfield, C. S., McGrath, P. J., & Finley, G. A. (2004) Risk factors for pain in children with severe cognitive impairments. *Developmental Medicine and Child Neurology 46*(6), 364–371.

Bremner, J. D., Staib, L., & Kaloupek, D. (1999). Neural correlates of exposure to traumatic pictures and sound in Vietnam combat veterans with and without posttraumatic stress disorder: a positron emission tomography study. *Biological Psychiatry, 45:* 806–816.

Brodal, A. (1980). *Neurological anatomy in relation to clinical medicine.* New York, NY: Oxford University Press.

Brodal, P. (1992). *The central nervous system: Structure and function.* New York, NY: Oxford University Press.

Bromberg, P. (1994). Speak! That I may see you. *Psychoanalytic Dialogues, 4,* 517–547.

Bromberg, P. (1998a). *Standing in the spaces: Essays on clinical process, trauma and dissociation.* Hillsdale, NJ: Analytic Press.

Bromberg, P. (1998b). Standing in the spaces: The multiplicity of self and the psycho-analytic relationship. In *Standing in the spaces: Essays on clinical process, trauma and dissociation* (pp. 267–290). Hillsdale, NJ: Analytic Press.

Bromberg, P. (1998c). On knowing one's patient inside out. In *Standing in the spaces: Essays on clinical process, trauma and dissociation* (pp. 127–146). Hillsdale, NJ: Analytic Press.

Butler, L. D. (2006). Normative dissociation. In R. A. Chefetz (Ed.), *Dissociative disorders: An expanding window into the psychobiology of the mind. Psychiatric Clinics of North America, 29*(1), (p. 45–62).

Buzsáki, G. (1996). The hippocampo–neocortical dialogue. *Cerebral Cortex, 6*, 81–92.

Carew, T. J., Hawkins, R. D., & Kandel, E. R. (1983). Differential classical conditioning of a defensive withdrawal reflex in *Aplysia californica. Science, 219*, 397–400.

Carpenter, M. D. (1991). *Cortex of neuroanatomy* (4th ed.). Baltimore, MD: Williams & Wilkins.

Chalmers, D. J. (1996). *The conscious mind: In search of a fundamental theory.* New York: Oxford University Press.

Chebat, D. R., Rainville, C., Kupers, R., & Ptito, M. 2007. Tactile–'visual' acuity of the tongue in early blind individuals. *Neuroreport, 18*(18), 1901–1904.

Chechik, G., Meilijson, I., & Ruppin, E. (1999). Neuronal regulation: A mechanism for synaptic pruning during brain maturation. *Neural Computation, 11*, 2061–2080.

Chefetz, R. A., & Bromberg, P. M. (2004). Talking with "me" and "not-me": A dialogue. *Contemporary Psychoanalysis, 40*(3), 409–464.

Clancy, R. (1998). Electroencephalography in the premature and full-term infant. In R. A. Poilin & W. W. Fox (Eds.), *Fetal and neonatal physiology* (pp. 2147–2165). W. B. Saunders.

Clark, D. D., & Sokoloff, L. (1999). Circulation and energy metabolism of the brain. In Siegel, G. J., Agranoff, B. W., Albers, R. W., Fisher, S. K., Uhler, M. D. (Eds.), *Basic Neurochemistry. Molecular, Cellular and Medical Aspects* (pp. 637–670). Philadelphia, PA: Lippincott–Raven.

Classen, C., Pain, C., Field, N. P., & Woods, P. (2006). Posttraumatic personality disorder: A reformulation of complex posttraumatic stress disorder and borderline personality disorder. In R. A. Chefetz (Ed.), *Dissociative disorders: An expanding window into the psychobiology of the mind. Psychiatric Clinics of North America, 29*(1), (87–112).

Closs, S. J., Barr, B., & Briggs, M. (2004). Cognitive status and analgesic provision in nursing home residents. *British Journal of General Practice 54*(509), 919–921.

Cobrin, G. M., & Abreu, M. T. (2005). Defects in mucosal immunity leading to Crohn's disease. *Immunological Reviews, 206*, 277–295.

Collins, D. R., Pelletier, J. G., & Paré, D. (2001). Slow and fast (gamma) neuronal oscillations in the perirhinal cortex and lateral amygdala. *Journal of Neurophysiology, 85*, 1661–1672.

Compton, A., & Coles, A. (2002). Multiple sclerosis. *Lancet, 359*(9313), 1221–1231.

Compton, A., & Coles, A. (2008). Multiple sclerosis. *Lancet, 372*(9648), 1502–1517.

Cooke, D. W., & Plotnick, L. (2008). Type 1 diabetes mellitus in pediatrics. *Pediatric Review, 29*(11), 374–84.

Corbett, D., & Wise, R. A. (1980). Intracranial self-stimulation in relation to the ascending dopaminergic systems of the midbrain: A moveable electrode mapping study. *Brain Research, 185*, 1–15.

Cotterill, R. M. (2001). Cooperation of the basal ganglia, cerebellum, sensory cerebrum and hippocampus: possible implications for cognition, consciousness, intelligence and creativity. *Progress in Neurobiology, 64*(1), 1–33.

Courchesne, E., & Allen, G. (1997). Prediction and preparation, fundamental functions of the cerebellum. *Learning & Memory, 4*(1), 1–35.

Courchesne, E., Townsend, J., Akshoomoff, N. A., Saitoh, O., Yeung-Courchesne, R., Lincoln, A. J., . . . Lau, L. (1994). Impairment in shifting attention in autistic and cerebellar patients. *Behavioral Neuroscience, 108*, 848–865.

Cozolino, L. (2002). *The neuroscience of psychotherapy: Building and rebuilding the human brain.* New York: W.W. Norton & Co.

Critchley, H. D., Corfield, D. R. & Chandler, M. D. (2000). Cerebral correlates of autonomic cardiovascular arousal: A functional neuroimaging investigation in humans. *Journal of Physiology, 523*, 259–27.

Damasio, A. R. (1998). Emotion in the perspective of an integrated nervous system. *Brain Research Reviews, 26*, 83–86.

Damasio, A. R. (1999). *The feeling of what happens.* New York, NY: Harcourt Inc.

Damasio, A. R. (2010). *Self comes to mind: constructing the conscious brain.* New York, NY: Pantheon Books.

Damasio, A. R., Eslinger, P. J., Damasio, H., Van Hoesen, G. W., & Cornell, S. (1985). Multimodal amnesic syndrome following bilateral temporal and basal forebrain damage. *Archives of Neurology, 42*(3), 252–259.

Dantzer, R. (2005). Somatization: A psychoneuroimmune perspective. *Pschoneuroendocrinology, 30*, 947–952.

De Charms, R. C., & Merzenich, M. M. (1996). Primary cortical representation of sounds by the coordination of action-potential timing. *Nature, 381*, 610–613.

De Rycke, L., Peene, I., Hoffman. I. E. A., Kruithof, E., Union, A., Meheus, L., . . . De Keyser, F. (2004). Rheumatoid factor and anticitrullinated protein antibodies in rheumatoid arthritis: diagnostic value, associations with radiological progression rate, and extra-articular manifestations. *Annals of Rheumatoid Disease, 63*, 1587–1593.

Derbyshire, S. W. G. (2006). Can fetuses feel pain? *British Medical Journal, 332*, 909–912.

Descartes, R. (1644). *Principia philosophiae (Principles of Philosophy)*, excerpted in vol. 1 of *The Philosophical Writings of Descartes*, ed. and trans. J. Cottingham, R. Stoothoff, D. Murdoch and A. Kenny, Cambridge: Cambridge University Press, 1984–91.

Dodd, J., & Role L. W. (1991). The autonomic nervous system. In E. R. Kandel, J. H. Schwartz, & T. M. Jessell (Eds.), *Principles of neural science* (3rd ed., pp. 761–775). New York, NY: Elsevier.

Doidge, N. (2007). *The brain that changes itself.* New York, NY: Penguin Books.

Dworkin, M. (2005). *EMDR and the relational imperative: The therapeutic relationship in EMDR treatment.* New York: Routledge.

Edelman, G. M. (1987). *Neural Darwinism: The theory of neuronal group selection.* New York, NY: Basic Books.

Edelman, G. M. (2006). Second nature: The transformation of knowledge. In *Second nature: Brain science and human knowledge* (pp. 142–157). New Haven, Connecticut: Yale University Press.

Eggermont, J. J. (1992). Neural interaction in cat primary auditory cortex. Dependence on recording depth, electrode separation, and age. *Journal of Neurophysiology, 68*, 1216–1228.

Elson, C. O., Cong, Y., Weaver, C. T., Schoeb, T. R., McClanahan, T. K., Fick, R. B., & Kastelein, R. A. (2007). Monoclonal anti–interleukin 23 reverses active colitis in a T cell-mediated model in mice. *Gastroenterology, 132*(7), 2359–2370.

Emde, R., Gaensbaure, T., & Harmon, R. (1976). Emotional expressions in infancy: A biobehavioral study (Monograph 37). *Psychological Issues, 10,* New York, NY: International Universities Press.

Engel, G. L. (1988). How much longer must medicine's science be bound by a seventeenth century world view? In K. L. White (Ed.), *The task of medicine: Dialogue at Wickenberg* (pp. 113–136). Menlo Park, CA: Henry J. Kaiser Foundation.

Engelmann, M., Landgraf, R., & Wotjak, C. (2004). The hypothalamic–neurohypophysial system regulates the hypothalamic–pituitary–adrenal axis under stress: An old concept revisited. *Frontiers of Neuroendocrinolpgy, 25*(3–4), 132–149.

Fairbairn, W. R. D. (1944). Endopsychic structure considered in terms of object-relationships. In *Psychoanalytic studies of the personality* (pp. 82–132). London, England: Routledge & Keegan Paul.

Fairbairn, W. R. D. (1952). *Psychoanalytic studies of the personality.* London, England: Routledge & Keegan Paul.

Fanselow, M. S., & Lester, L. S. (1988). A functional behavioristic approach to aversively motivated behavior: Predatory imminent as a determinant of the topography of defensive behavior. In R. C. Bolles & M. D. Beecher (Eds.), *Evolution and learning.* Hillsdale, New Jersey: Erlbaum.

Federn, P. (1943). Psychoanalysis of psychosis. *Psychoanalytic Quarterly, 17,* 3–19, 246–257, 480–487.

Federn, P. (1947). Principles of psychotherapy in latent schizophrenics. *American Journal of Psychotherapy, 1,* 129–144.

Federn, P. (1952). *Ego psychology and the psychoses.* New York, NY: Basic Books.

Feldt, K. S., Ryden, M. B., & Miles, S. (1998). Treatment of pain in cognitively impaired compared with cognitively intact older patients with hip-fracture. *Journal of the American Geriatric Society, 46*(9), 1079–1085.

Felten, D. L., Hallman, H., & Jonsson, G. (1982). Evidence for a neurotrophic role of noradrenalin neurons in the postnatal development of rat cerebral cortex. *Journal of Neurocytology, 11,* 119–135.

Ferenczi, S. (1930). Notes and fragments II. In M. Balint (Ed.), *Final contributions to the problems and methods of psychoanalysis* (pp. 219–231). New York, NY: Brunner/Mazel.

Fernandez, T., Harmony, T., Silva, J., Galin, L., Diaz–Comas, L., Bosch, J., . . . Marosi, E. (1998). Relationship of specific EEG frequencies at specific brain areas with performance. *Neuroreport, 9*(16), 3680–3687.

Ferrell, B. A., Ferrell, B. R. & Rivera, L. (1995) Pain in cognitively impaired nursing home patients. *Journal of Pain and Symptom Management, 10*(8), 591–598.

Forster, M. C., Pardiwala, A., & Calthorpe, D. (2000). Analgesia requirements following hip fracture in the cognitively impaired. *Injury, 31*(6), 435–436.

Freud, A. (1936). The ego and the mechanisms of defense. *The writings of Anna Freud* (Vol. 2). New York, NY: International Universities Press.

Freud, A. (1963). The concept of developmental lines. *The Psychoanalytic Study of the Child, 18,* 245–265.

Freud, S. (1954/1895). A project for a scientific psychology. In James Strachey (Ed.), *The standard edition of the complete psychological works of Sigmund Freud* (Vol. 1, p. 283–392). London, England: The Hogarth Press.

Frewen, P. A., & Lanius, R. A. (2006). Neurobiology of dissociation: Unity and disunity in mind–body–brain. In R. A. Chefetz (Ed.), Dissociative disorders: An expanding window into the psychobiology of the mind. *Psychiatric Clinics of North America, 29*(1): 113–128.

Fries, E., Hesse, J., Hellhammer, J., & Hellhammer, D. H. (2005). A new view on hypocortisolism. *Psychoneuroendocrinology, 30*(10), 1010–1016.

Gallese, V. (2003). The roots of empathy: The shared manifold hypothesis and the neural basis of intersubjectivity. *Psychopathology, 36,* 171–180.

Gazzaniga, M. S. (1970). *The bisected brain.* New York, NY: Appleton–Century Crofts.

Gazzaniga, M. S. (1976). The biology of human memory. In M. Rosenzweig & M. Bennet (Eds.), *Neural mechanisms of learning and memory* (pp. 57–66). Cambridge, MA: MIT Press.

Gazzaniga, M. S. (1989). Organization of the human brain. *Science, 245,* 947–95.

Gazzaniga, M. S. (1998). The split-brain revisited. *Scientific American, 279,* 50–55.

Gazzaniga, M. S. (2000). Cerebral specialization and interhemispheric communication: Does the corpus callosum enable the human condition? *Brain, 123,* 1293–1326.

Gazzaniga, M. S., & LeDoux, J. (1978). *The integrated mind.* New York, NY: Plenum Press.

Gazzaniga, M. S., LeDoux, J., & Wilson, D. H. (1977). Language praxis and the right hemisphere: Clues to some mechanisms of consciousness. *Neurology, 27,* 1144–1147.

Glover, E. (1932). A psycho-analytical approach to the classification of mental disorders. In *On the early development of the mind* (pp. 161–186). New York, NY: International Universities Press.

Goleman, D. (1995). *Emotional intelligence.* New York, NY: Bantam Books.

Gomez–Pinilla, F., Choi, J., & Ryba, E. A. (1999). Visual input regulates the expression of basic fibroblast growth factor and its receptor. *Neuroscience, 88,* 1051–1058.

Gray, C. M. (1994). Synchronous oscillations in neuronal systems: Mechanisms and functions. *Journal of Computational Neuroscience, 1,* 11–38.

Gray, C. M., & Singer, W. (1989). Stimulus-specific neuronal oscillations in orientation columns of cat visual cortex. *Proc. National Academy of Sciences, USA, 86,* 1698–1702.

Grossberg, S. (1976). Adaptive pattern classification and universal recoding: Part 1. Parallel development and coding of neural feature detectors. *Biological Cybernetics, 23,* 121–134.

Haith, M. M., Bergman, T., & Moore, M. (1979). Eye contact and face scanning in early infancy. *Science, 218,* 179–181.

Hammer, M., & Menzel, R. (1995). Learning and memory in the honeybee. *Journal of Neuroscience, 15,* 1617–1630.

Hari, R., Salmelin, S., Makela, J. P., Salenius, S., & Helle, M. (1997). Magnetoencephalographic cortical rhythms. *International Journal of Psychophysiology, 26,* 51–62.

Hawkins, R. D., Abrams, D. W., Carew, T. J., & Kandel, E. R. (1983). A cellular mechanism of classical conditioning in Aplysia: Activity-dependant application of pre-synaptic facilitation. *Science, 219,* 400–405.

Hebb, D. O. (1949). *The organization of behavior: A neuropsychological theory.* New York, NY: Wiley.

Heim, C., Ehlert, U., & Hellhammer, D. H. (2000). The potential role of hypocortisolism in the pathophysiology of stress-related bodily disorders. *Psychoneuroendocrinology, 25*, 1–35.

Henry, J. P., Haviland, M. G., Cummings, M. A., Anderson, D. L., MacMurray, F. P., McGhee, W. H., & Hubbard, R. W. (1992). Shared neuroendocrine patterns of post-traumatic-stress disorder and alexithymia. *Psychosomatic Medicine, 54*, 407–415.

Herman, J. L. (1992). *Trauma and recovery*. New York, NY: Basic Books.

Herman, J. L., Perry, J. C., & van der Kolk, B. A. (1989). Childhood trauma in borderline personality disorder. *American Journal of Psychiatry, 146*, 49–495.

Herrmann, C. S., Munk, M. H. J., & Engel, A. K. (2004). Cognitive functions of gamma band activity: Memory match and utilization. *Trends in Cognitive Sciences, 8*(8), 347–355.

Hess, E. H. (1975). The role of pupil size in communication. *Scientific American, 233*, 110–119.

Hobson, A. (2009). Prologue. In S. Laureys & G. Tononi (Eds.), *The neurology of consciousness* (pp. xi–xii). New York, NY: Elsevier, Academic Press.

Hokama, Y., Campora, C. E., Hara, C., Kuribayashi, T., Huynh, D. L., & Yabusaki, K. (2009). Anticardiolipin antibodies in the sera of patients with diagnosed chronic fatigue syndrome. *Journal of Clinical Laboratory Analysis, 23*, 210–212.

Hollrigel, G. S., Chen, K., Baram, T. Z., & Soltesz, I. (1998). The pro-convulsant actions of corticotrophin-releasing hormone in the hippocampus of infant rats. *Neuroscience, 84*, 71–79.

Horgas, A. L., & Tsai, P. F. (1998). Analgesic drug prescription and use in cognitively impaired nursing home residents. *Nursing Research, 47*(4), 235–242.

Huang, Z. J., Kirkwood, A., Pizzorusso, T., Porciatti, V., Morales, B., Bear, M. F., . . . Tonegawa, S. (1999). BDNF regulates the maturation of inhibition and the critical period of plasticity in mouse visual cortex. *Cell, 98*, 739–755.

Hugdahl, K. (1995). Classical conditioning and implicit learning. In R. J. Davidson & K. Hugdahl (Eds.), *Brain Asymmetry* (pp. 235–267). Cambridge, MA: MIT Press.

Huygen, F. J., de Bruijn, A. G., Klein, J., & Zijlstra, F. J. (2001). Neuroimmune alterations in the complex regional pain syndrome. *European Journal of Pharmacology, 429*(1–3), 101–113.

Iglesias, A., Bauer, J., Litzenburger, T., Schubart, A., & Linington, C. (2001). T- and B-cell responses to myelin oligodendrocyte glycoprotein in experimental autoimmune encephalomyelitis and multiple sclerosis. *Glia, 36*(2), 220–234.

Iglesias, P., Dévora, O., García, J., Tajada, P., García–Arévalo, C., & Díez, J. J. (2009). Severe hyperthyroidism: Aetiology, clinical features and treatment outcome. *Clinical Endocrinology, 72*(4), 551–7.

Ishai, A., Ungerleider, L. G., Martin, A., Schouten, J. L., & Haxby, J. V. (1999). Distributed representation of objects in the human ventral visual pathway. *Proceedings of the National Academy of Sciences (USA), 96*, 9379–9384.

Iversen, S. D. (1997). Brain dopamine systems and behavior. In Iversen, S. D. and Snyder, S. H. (Eds.), *Drugs, neurotransmitters and behavior: Handbook of psychopharmacology*. New York, NY: Plenum.

Jackson, J. H. (1958). On localization [original work published in 1869]. In *Selected writings* (Vol. 2). New York, NY: Basic Books.

Jacob, F. (1982). *The possible and the actual*. New York, NY: Pantheon.

James, W. (1890). *The Principles of Psychology*. Cambridge: Harvard University Press.

Janet, P. (1907). *The major symptoms of hysteria*. London, England, & New York, NY: Macmillan.

Janet, P. (1911). *L'etat mental des hysteriques [The mental state of the hysteric]* (2nd Ed.). Paris: Alcan.

Janet, P. (1925). *Psychological healing* (Vols. 1–2; C. Paul & E. Paul, Trans.) [original work published in 1919]. New York, NY: Macmillan.

Jeffreys, J. G. R., Traub, R. D., & Whittington, M. A. (1996). Neuronal networks for induced "40 Hz" rhythms. *Trends in Neurosciences, 19*, 202–208.

Johnston, C. C., Collinge, J. M., Henderson, S. J., & Anand, K. J. S. (1997). A cross-sectional survey of pain and pharmacological analgesia in Canadian neonatal intensive care units. *Clinical Journal of Pain, 13*(4), 308–312.

Jokisch, D., & Jensen, O. (2007). Modulation of gamma and alpha activity during a working memory task engaging the dorsal or ventral stream. *Journal of Neuroscience, 27*(12), 3224–3251.

Joliot, M., Ribary, U., & Llinas, R. (1994). Human oscillatory brain activity near 40 Hz coexists with cognitive temporal binding. *Proceedings of the National Academy of Sciences USA, 91*, 11748–11751.

Kalin, N. H., Shelton, S. E., & Lynn, D. E. (1995). Opiate systems in mother and infant primates coordinate intimate contact during reunion. *Psychoneuroendocrinology, 20*, 735–742.

Kandel, E. (1989). Genes, nerve cells, and the remembrance of things past. *Journal of Neuropsychiatry, 1*(2), 103–125.

Kandel, E. (1998). A new intellectual framework for psychiatry. *The American Journal of Psychiatry, 155*, 457–469.

Kandel, E. (2000). Cellular mechanisms of learning and the biological basis of individuality. In E. Kandel, J. Schwartz, & T. Jessell (Eds.), *Principles of neural science* (4th ed., pp. 1247–1279). New York, NY: Elsevier.

Kandel, E. R. (1991a). Brain and behavior. In E. R. Kandel, J. H. Schwartz, & T. M. Jessell (Eds.), *Principles of neural science* (3rd ed., pp. 5–17). New York, NY: Elsevier.

Kandel, E. R. (1991b). Transmitter release. In E. R. Kandel, J. H. Schwartz, & T. M. Jessell (Eds.), *Principles of neural science* (3rd ed., pp. 195–212). New York, NY: Elsevier.

Kandel, E. R. (2006). *In search of memory: The emergence of a new science of mind*. New York, NY: W. W. Norton & Co.

Kandel, E. R., Brunelli, M., Byrne, J., & Castellucci, V. (1976). A common presynaptic locus for the synaptic changes underlying short-term habituation and sensitization of the gill withdrawal reflex in Aplysia. *Biology, 40*, 465–582.

Kandel, E. R., Siegelbaum, S. A., & Schwartz, J. H. (1991). Synaptic transmission. In E. R. Kandel, J. H. Schwartz, & T. M. Jessell (Eds.), *Principles of neural science* (3rd ed., pp. 123–134). New York, NY: Elsevier.

Katz, B. (1959a). Nature of the nerve impulse. *Review of Modern Physics, 31*, 466–474.

Katz, B. (1959b). Mechanisms of synaptic transmission. *Review of Modern Physics, 31*, 524–531.

Katz, B. (1971). Quantal mechanism of neural transmitter release. *Science, 173*, 123–126.

Klein, M. (1946). Notes on some schizoid mechanism. *International Journal of Psycho Analysis, 27*, 99–110.

Klimesch, W. (1999). EEG alpha and theta oscillations reflect cognitive and memory performance: A review and analysis. *Brain Research Reviews 29*(2–3), 169–195.

Koester, J. (1991). Membrane potential. In E. R. Kandel, J. H. Schwartz, & T. M. Jessell (Eds.), *Principles of neural science* (3rd ed., pp. 81–94). New York, NY: Elsevier.

Koh, J. L., Fanurik, D., Harrison, R. D., Schmitz, M. L., & Norvell, D. (2004). Analgesia following surgery in children with and without cognitive impairment. *Pain, 111*(3), 239–244.

Kojima, K., Kaneko, T., & Yasuda, K. (2004). A novel method of cultivating cardiac myocytes in agarose microchamber chips for studying cell synchronization. *Journal of Nanobiotechnology, 2*(9), 1–4.

Kristeva–Feige, R., Feige, B., Makeig, S., Ross, B., & Elbert, T. (1993). Oscillatory brain activity during a motor task. *Neuroreport, 4*, 1291–1294.

Krystal, H. (1988). *Integration and self-healing: Affect-trauma-alexithymia.* Hillsdale, NJ: Analytic Press.

Kupfermann, I. (1991a). Hypothalamus and limbic system: Peptidergic neurons, homeostasis, and emotional behavior. In E. R. Kandel, J. H. Schwartz, & T. M. Jessell (Eds.), *Principles of neural science* (3rd ed., pp. 735–749). New York, NY: Elsevier.

Kupfermann, I. (1991b). Localization of higher cognitive and affective functions: The association cortices. In E. R. Kandel, J. H. Schwartz, & T. M. Jessell (Eds.), *Principles of neural science* (3rd ed., pp. 823–838). New York, NY: Elsevier.

Kupfermann, I., Castellucci, V., Pinsker, H., & Kandel, E.R. (1970). Neuronal mechanisms of habituation and dishabituation of the gill-withdrawal reflex in Aplysia. *Science, 167*, 1745–1748.

Lampl-de-Groot, J. (1981). Notes on "multiple personality." *Psychoanalytic Quarterly, 50*, 614–624.

Lanius, R. A., Bluhm, R., & Lanius, U. (2007). Posttraumatic stress disorder symptom provocation and neuroimaging. In E. Vermetten, M. J. Dorahy, & D. Spiegel (Eds.), *Traumatic dissociation: Neurobiology and treatment* (pp. 191–217). Washington, DC: American Psychiatric Publishing.

Lanius, R. A., Williamson, P. C., Bluhm, R. L., Densmore, M., Boksman, K., Neufeld, R. W. J., . . . Menon, R. S. (2005). Functional connectivity of dissociative responses in posttraumatic stress disorder: A functional magnetic resonance imaging investigation. *Biological Psychiatry, 57*, 873–84.

Lanius, R. A., Williamson, P. C., & Densmore, M. (2001). Neural correlates of traumatic memories in posttraumatic stress disorder: A functional MRI investigation. *American Journal of Psychiatry, 158*, 1920–1922.

Lanius, R. A., Williamson, P. C., & Hopper, J. (2003). Recall of emotional states in posttraumatic stress disorder: An fMRI investigation. *Biological Psychiatry, 53*, 204–210.

Larsell, O., & Jansen, J. (1972). *The comparative anatomy and histology of the cerebellum* (Vol. 3). Minneapolis, MN: University of Minnesota Press.

Lashley, K. S. (1950). In search of the engram. In *Society of Experimental Biology Symposium, No. 4, Psychological Mechanisms in Animal Behavior* (pp. 478–505). London, England: Cambridge University Press.

Laureys, S., Faymonville, M. E., Luxen, A., Lamy, M., Franck, G., & Maquet, P. (2000). Restoration of thalamocortical connectivity after recovery from persistent vegetative state. *Lancet, 355*, 1790–1791.

LeDoux, J. (1986). Sensory systems and emotions. *Integrative Psychiatry, 4*, 237–248.

LeDoux, J. (1992). Emotions and the limbic system concept. *Concepts in Neuroscience, 2*, 169–199.

LeDoux, J. (1994). Emotion, memory and the brain. *Scientific American, 270,* 50–57.

LeDoux, J. (1996). *The emotional brain: The mysterious underpinnings of emotional life.* New York, NY: Simon & Schuster.

LeDoux, J. (2002). *Synaptic self: How our brains become who we are.* New York, NY: Viking.

LeDoux, J. (2003). The self: Clues from the brain. *Annals of the New York Academy of Sciences, 1001,* 295–304.

Lee, S. J., Ralston, H. J. P., Drey, E. A., Partridge, J. C., & Rosen, M. A. (2005) Fetal pain: A systematic multidisciplinary review of the evidence. *Journal of the American Medical Association, 294*(8), 947–954.

Legakis, I., Petroyianni, V., Saramantis, A., & Tolis, G. (2001). Elevated prolactin to cortisol ratio and polyclonal autoimmune activation in Hashimoto's thyroiditis. *Hormonal Metabolic Research, 10,* 585–589.

Leiner, H. C., Leiner, A. L., & Dow, R. S. (1986). Does the cerebellum contribute to mental skills? *Behavioral Neuroscience, 100,* 443–454.

Leiner, H. C., Leiner, A. L., & Dow, R. S. (1991). The human cerebro–cerebellar system: Its computing, cognitive and language skills. *Behavioral Brain Research, 44,* 113–128.

Liberzon, I., Taylor, S. F. and Amdur, R. (1999). Brain activation in PTSD in response to trauma related stimuli. *Biological Psychiatry, 45,* 817–826.

Liu, D., Diorio, J., Day, J. C., Francis, D. D., & Meany, M. J. (2000). Maternal care, hippocampal synaptogenesis and cognitive development in rats. *Nature Neuroscience, 3,* 799–806.

Llinas, R. R. (1987). "Mindedness" as a functional state of the brain. In C. Blackmore & S. A. Greenfield (Eds.), *Mind waves* (pp. 339–358). Oxford, England: Basil Blackwell.

Llinas, R. R. (1988). The intrinsic electrophysiological properties of mammalian neurons: Insights into central nervous system function. *Science, 242,* 1654–1664.

Llinas, R. R. (2001). *I of the vortex. From neurons to self.* Cambridge, Massachusetts: The MIT Press.

Llinas, R. R., Grace, A. A., & Yarom, Y. (1991). In vitro neurons in mammalian cortical layer 4 exhibit intrinsic activity in the 10 to 50 Hz frequency range. *Proceedings of the National Academy of Sciences of the United States of America, 88,* 897–901.

Llinas, R. R., Leznik, E., & Urbano, F. J. (2003). Temporal binding via cortical coincidence detection of specific and nonspecific thalamo–cortical inputs: A voltage dependent high imaging study in mouse brain slices. *Proceedings of the National Academy of Sciences, 99*(1), 449–454.

Llinas, R. R., & Pare, D. (1991). Of dreaming and wakefulness. *Neuroscience, 44,* 521–535.

Llinas, R. R., & Ribary, U. (1993). Coherent 40 Hz oscillation characterizes dream state in humans. *Proceedings of the National Academy of Sciences, USA, 90,* 2078–2081.

Llinas, R. R., & Ribary, U. (2001). Consciousness and the brain: The thalamo–cortical dialogue in health and disease. *Annals of the New York Academy of Sciences, 929,* 166–175.

Llinas, R. R., & Sotelo, C. (1992). *The cerebellum revisited.* New York, NY: Springer Publishing.

Loewenstein, R. J. (2007). Dissociative identity disorder: Issues in the iatrogenesis controversy. In E. Vermetten, M. J. Dorahy, & D. Spiegel (Eds.), *Traumatic dissociation: Neurobiology and treatment* (pp. 275–299). Washington, DC: American Psychiatric Publishing.

Lyons, G., Sanabria, D., Vatakis, A., & Spence, C. (2006). The modulation of crossmodal integration by unimodal perceptual grouping: A visuotactile apparent motion study. *Experimental Brain Research, 174*(3), 510–516.

Macaluso, E., & Driver, J. (2005). Multisensory spatial interactions: A window onto functional integration in the human brain. *Trends in Neurosciences, 28*(5), 264–271.

Maes, M., Libbrecht, I., Van Hunsel, F., Lin, A. H., De Clerck, L., Stevens, W., . . . Neels, H. (1999). The immune–inflammatory pathophysiology of fibromyalgia: Increased serum soluble gp130, the common signal transducer protein of various neurotrophic cytokines. *Psychoneuroendocrinology, 24*, 371–383.

Mahler, M. S. (1967). On human symbiosis and the vicissitudes of individuation. In *The selected papers of Margaret S. Mahler* (Vol. 2, p. 77–97). New York, NY: Jason Aronson.

Mahler, M. S. (1972). On the first three subphases of the separation–individuation process. In *The selected papers of Margaret S. Mahler* (Vol. 2, p. 119–130). New York, NY: Jason Aronson.

Male, D., Brostoff, J., Roth, D., & Roitt, I. (2006). *Immunology* (7th ed.) New York, NY: Elsevier.

Malviya, S., Voepel–Lewis, T., Tait, A., Merkel, S., Lauer, A., Munro, H., & Farley, F. (2001). Pain management in children with and without cognitive impairment following spine fusion surgery. *Pediatric Anesthesia, 11*(4), 453.

Martin, J. H. (1991). Coding and processing of sensory information. In E. R. Kandel, J. H. Schwartz, & T. M. Jessell (Eds.), *Principles of neural science* (3rd ed., pp. 329–366). New York: Elsevier.

Mason, J. W., Giller, E. L., Kosten, T. R., Ostroff, R., & Harkness, L. (1986). Urinary free cortisol levels in post traumatic stress disorder patients. *Journal of Nervous Mental Disorders, 174*, 145–149.

Mastorakos, G., Karoutsou, E. I., & Mizamtsidi, M. (2006). Corticotropin releasing hormone and the immune/inflammatory response. *European Journal of Endocrinology, 155*, 77–84.

McClelland, J. L. (1979). On the time relations of mental processes: An examination of systems of processes in cascade. *Psychological Review, 86*, 287–330.

McClelland, J. L. (1994). The organization of memory: A parallel distributed processing perspective. *Revue Nurologique, 150*(8–9), 570–579.

McClelland, J. L. (1996). Role of the hippocampus in learning and memory: A computational analysis. In T. Ono, B. L. McNaughton, S. Molitchnikoff, E. T. Rolls, & H. Nichijo (Eds.), *Perception, memory and emotion: Frontier in neuroscience* (pp. 601–613). Oxford: Elsevier Science.

McClelland, J. L., McNaughton, B. L., & O'Reilly, R. C. (1995). Why there are complementary learning systems in the hippocampus and neocortex: Insights from the successes and failures of connectionist models of learning and memory. *Psychological Review, 102*, 419–457.

McLachlan, S. M., & Rappaport, B. (1992). The molecular biology of thyroid peroxidase: Cloning, expression and role as autoantigen in autoimmune thyroid disease. *Endocrine Review, 13*, 192–206.

Mellor, D. J., Diesch, T. J., Gunn, A. J., & Bennet, L. (2005). The importance of "awareness" for understanding fetal pain. *Brain Research Reviews, 49*, 455–471.

Merker, B. (2007). Consciousness without a cerebral cortex: A challenge for neuroscience and medicine. *Behavioral and Brain Sciences, 30*, 63–134.

Montgomery, S. M., Buzsáki, G. (2007). Gamma oscillations dynamically couple hippocampal CA3 and CA1 regions during memory task performance. *Proceedings of the National Academy of Sciences, 104*(36), 14495–14500.

Moreno, J. L. (1934). *Who shall survive? A new approach to the problems of human interrelations.* Washington, DC: Nervous and Mental Disease Publishing Co.

Moreno, J. L. (1943). Sociometry and the control order. *Sociometry, 6*(3), 299–344.

Morin, A. (2006). Levels of consciousness and self-awareness: A comparison and integration of various neurocognitive views. *Consciousness and Cognition, 15*, 358–371.

Morris, C. D., Bransford, J. D., & Franks, J. J. (1977). Levels of processing versus transfer appropriate processing. *Journal of Verbal Learning and Verbal Behavior, 16,* 519–533.

Mulligan, N. W., & Lozito, J. P. (2006). An asymmetry between memory encoding and retrieval. *Psychological Science, 17*(1), 7–11.

Murthy, V. N., & Fetz, E. E. (1996). Synchronization of neurons during local field potential oscillations in sensorimotor cortex of awake monkeys. *Journal of Neurophysiology, 76,* 3968–3982.

Myers, C. S. (1940). *Shell Shock in France, 1914–1918.* Cambridge: Cambridge University Press.

Myers, L. B., & Bulich, L. A. (2005). *Anesthesia for fetal intervention and surgery.* Hamilton, British Columbia: Decker.

Nadel, L., & Moscovitch, M. (1998). Hippocampal contributions to cortical plasticity. *Neuropharmacology, 37,* 431–439.

Nauta, W. J . H., & Domesick, V. B. (1982). Neural associations of the limbic system. In A. L. Beckman (Ed.), *The neural basis of behavior* (pp. 175–206). New York, NY: SP Medical and Scientific Books.

Nijenhuis, E. R. S., van der Hart, O., & Steele, K. (2002). The emerging psychobiology of trauma related dissociation and dissociative disorders. In H. D'Haenen, J. A. den Boer, & P. Willner (Eds.), *Biological psychiatry* (pp. 1079–1098). London, England: Wile.

Noback, C. R., & Demarest, R. J. (1981). *The human nervous system: Basic principles of neurobiology* (3rd ed.). New York, NY: McGraw–Hill.

Ogden, T. H. (1982). *Projective identification & psychotherapeutic technique.* New York, NY: Jason Aronson.

O'Keefe, J., & Dostrovsky, J. (1971). The hippocampus as a spatial map: Preliminary evidence from unit activity in the freely-moving rat. *Brain Research, 34*(1), 171–175.

O'Keefe, J., & Nadel, L. (1978). *The hippocampus as a cognitive map.* London, England: Oxford University Press.

Orlinsky, D. E., & Howard, K. I. (1986). Process and outcome in psychotherapy. In S. L. Garfield & A. E. Bergin (Eds.), *Handbook of psychotherapy and behavior change* (3rd ed., pp. 311–381). New York, NY: Wiley.

Orr, S. P., McNally, R. J., & Rosen, G. M. (2004). Psychophysiological reactivity: Implications for conceptualizing in PTSD. In G. M. Rosen (Ed.), *Posttraumatic stress disorder: Issues and controversies* (pp. 101–126). New York, NY: John Wiley & Sons.

Ortega–Hernandez, O. D., & Schoenfeld, Y. (2009). Infection, vaccination, and autoantibodies in chronic fatigue syndrome, cause or coincidence? *Annals of the New York Academy of Science, 1173,* 600–609.

Osipova, D., Takamisha, A., Oostenveld, R., Fernandez, G., Maris, E., & Jansen, O. (2006). Theta and gamma oscillations predict encoding and retrieval of declarative memory. *Journal of Neuroscience, 26*(28), 7523–7531.

Palm, G. (1990). Cell assemblies as a guideline for brain research. *Concepts in Neuroscience, 1,* 133–147.

Panksepp, J. (1998). *Affective neuroscience: The foundations of human animal emotions.* New York, NY: Oxford University Press.

Papassotiropoulos, A., Wollmer, M. A., Aguzzi, A., Hock, C., Nitsch, R. M., & de Quervin, D. J. (2005). *Human Molecular Genetics, 14*(15), 2241–2246.

Parmelee, P. A. (1996) Pain in cognitively impaired older persons. *Clinics in Geriatric Medicine 12*(3), 473–487.

Pavlides, C., & Winson, J. (1989). Influences of hippocampal place cell firing in the awake state on the activity of these cells during subsequent sleep episodes. *Journal of Neuroscience, 9,* 2907–2918.

Pavlov, I. P. (1927). *Conditioned Reflexes.* Oxford: Humphrey Milford.

Peigneux, P., Laureys, S., Fuchs, S., Collette, F., Perrin, F., Reggers, J., . . . Maquet, P. (2004). Are spatial memories strengthened in the human hippocampus during slow wave sleep? *Neuron, 44,* 535–545.

Peterson, S. E., Fox, P. T., Posner, M. I., Mintun, M., & Raichle, M. E. (1989). Positron emission tomographic studies of the processing of single words. *Journal of Cognitive Neuroscience, 1,* 153–170.

Plihal, W., & Born, J. (1997). Effects of early and late nocturnal sleep on declarative and procedural memory. *Journal of Cognitive Neuroscience, 9*(4), 534–547.

Porges, S. W. (1997). Emotion: An evolutionary by-product of the neural regulation of the autonomic nervous system. *Annals of the New York Academy of Sciences, 807,* 62–77.

Porges, S. W. (2001). The polyvagal theory: Phylogenetic substrates of a social nervous system. *International Journal of Psychophysiology, 42,* 123–146.

Porges, S. W. (2011). The early development of the autonomic nervous system provides a neural platform for social behavior: A polyvagal perspective. *Infant Child Development, 20*(1), 106–118.

Porter, F. L., & Anand, K. J. S. (1998). Epidemiology of pain in neonates. *Research & Clinical Forums, 20*(4), 9–16.

Posner, J. B., & Plum, F. (2007). *Plum and Posner's diagnosis of stupor and coma* (4th ed.). New York, NY: Oxford University Press.

Prince, S. E., Daselaar, S. M., & Cabeza, R. (2005). Neural correlates of relational memory: Successful encoding and retrieval of semantic and perceptual associations. *Journal of Neuroscience, 25*(5), 1203–1210.

Putnam, F. (1988). The switch processes in multiple personality disorder and other state-change disorders. *Dissociation, 1,* 24–32.

Putnam, F. (1995a). Resolved: Multiple personality disorder is an individually and socially created artifact. *Journal of the American Academy of Child and Adolescent Psychiatry, 34,* 960–962.

Putnam, F. (1995b). Resolved: Multiple personality disorder is an individually and socially created artifact. Negative rebuttal. *Journal of the American Academy of Child and Adolescent Psychiatry, 34,* 963.

Pynoos, R. S., & Nader, K. (1988). Children's memory and proximity to violence. *Journal of the American Academy of Child and Adolescent Psychiatry, 27,* 236–244.

Rahman, A., & Isenberg, D. A. (2008). Review article: Systemic lupus erythematosus. *New England Journal of Medicine, 358*(9), 929–939.

Raichle, M. E. (2006). The brain's dark energy. *Science, 314*, 1249–1250.

Raichle, M. E. (2009). A paradigm shift in functional brain imaging. *The Journal of Neuroscience, 29*(41), 12729–12734.

Ramachandran, V. S. (1995). Anosognosia in parietal lobe syndrome. *Consciousness & Cognition, 4*, 22–51.

Ramachandran, V. S. (2000). Mirror neurons and imitation learning as the driving force behind "the great leap forward" in human evolution. *Edge, 69.* Retrieved from http://www. edge.org/3rd_culture/ramachandran/ramachandran_p1.html

Ramachandran, V. S., & Blakeslee, S. (1998). *Phantoms in the brain.* New York, NY: Quill/HarperCollins.

Ramon y Cajal, S. (1899). *Textura del systemo nervioso del hombre y de los Vertebrados* [Texture of the nervous system of man and vertebrates]. Madrid, Spain: N. Moya.

Rasch, B., Buchel, C., Gais, S., & Born, J. (2007). Odor cues during slow wave sleep prompt declarative memory consolidation. *Science, 315*(5817), 1426–1429.

Reinders, A. A. T. S., Nijenhuis, E. R. S., Paans, A. M. J., Korf, J., Willemsen, A. T. M., & . . . den Boer, J. A. (2003). One brain, two selves. *NeuroImage, 20,* 2119–2125.

Reinders, A. A. T. S., Nijenhuis, E. R. S., Quak, J., Korf, J., Haaksma, J., Paans, A. M. J., den Boer, J. A. (2006). Psychobiological characteristics of dissociative identity disorder: A symptom provocation study. *Biological Psychiatry, 60,* 730–740.

Reiser, M. (1994). *Memory in mind and brain: What dream imagery reveals.* New Haven, CT: Yale University Press.

Rizzolatti, G., & Craighero, L. (2004). The mirror-neuron system. *Annual Review of Neuroscience, 27,* 169–192.

Romanski, L. M., Tian, B., Fritz, J., Mishkin, M., Goldman–Rakic, P. S., & Rauschecker, J. P. (1999). Dual streams of auditory afferents target multiple domains in the primate prefrontal cortex. *Nature Neuroscience, 2,* 113–1136.

Rosenthal, D. M. (2002). How many kinds of consciousness? *Consciousness and Cognition, 11,* 653–65.

Rothbart, M. K., Taylor, S. B., & Tucker, D. M. (1989). Right-sided facial asymmetry in infant emotional expression. *Neuropsychologia, 27,* 675–687.

Rothwell, N. J. (1999). Annual review prize lecture cytokines killers in the brain? *Journal of Physiology, 514*(Pt. 1), 3–17.

Rumelhart, & McClelland. (1986). *Parallel distributed processing: Explorations in the microstructure of cognition,* Vol. 1. Cambridge, Massachusetts: The MIT Press.

Sander, L. (1977). The regulation of exchange in the infant caretaker system and some aspects of the context–content relationship. In M. Lewis & L. Rosenblum (Eds.), *Interaction, conservation, and the development of language* (pp. 133–156). New York, NY: Wiley.

Sanders, P., & Korf, J. (2008). Neuroaetiology of chronic fatigue syndrome: An overview. *World Journal of Biological Psychiatry, 9*(3), 165–171.

Sands, S. H. (1997). Protein or foreign body? Reply to commentaries. *Psychoanalytic Dialogues, 7,* 691–706.

Saravanan, P., & Dayan, C. M. (2001). Thyroid autoantibodies. *Endocrinological Metabolism Clinics of North America, 30*(2), 315–335.

Scalaidhe, S. P., Wilson, F. A. W., & Goldman–Rakic, P. S. (1997). Areal segregation of face-processing neurons in prefrontal cortex. *Science, 278,* 1135–1138.

Schacter, D. L., Chiu, C.-Y. P., & Ochsner, K. N. (1993). Implicit memory: A selective review. *Annual Reviews of Neuroscience, 16,* 159–182.

Schore, A. N. (1994). *Affect regulation and the origin of the self: The neurobiology of emotional development.* Mahwah, NJ: Erlbaum.

Schore, A. N. (2001a). The effects of a secure attachment relationship on right brain development, affect regulation and infant mental health. *Infant Mental Health Journal, 22*(1–2), 7–66.

Schore, A. N. (2001b). The effects of early relational trauma on right brain development and infant mental health. *Infant Mental Health Journal, 22*(1–2), 201–269.

Schore, A. N. (2003a). *Affect dysregulation and disorders of the self.* New York, NY: W. W. Norton & Co.

Schore, A. N. (2003b). *Affect regulation and the repair of the self.* New York, NY: W. W. Norton & Co.

Schwartz, J. H. (1991). Chemical messengers: Small molecules and peptides. In E. R. Kandel, J. H. Schwartz, & T. M. Jessell (Eds.), *Principles of neural science* (3rd ed., pp. 213–224). New York, NY: Elsevier.

Schwartz, R. C. (1995). *Internal family systems therapy.* New York, NY: Guilford Press.

Searles, H. F. (1977). Dual and multi-identity processes in borderline ego functioning. In P. Hartocollis (Ed.), *Borderline personality disorders* (pp. 441–455). New York, NY: International Universities Press.

Sederberg, P. B., Schulze–Bonhage, A., Madsen, J. R., Bromfield, E. B., Litt, B., Brandt, A., & Kahana, M. J. (2007). Gamma oscillations distinguished true from false memories. *Psychological Science, 18*(11), 927–932.

Selemon, L., Goldmanrakic, P., & Tamminga, C. (1995). Prefrontal cortex and working memory. *American Journal of Psychiatry, 152*(1), 5–16.

Shapiro, F. (1995). Eye movement sensitization and reprocessing: Basic principles, protocols, and procedures (1st ed.). New York, NY: Guilford Press.

Shapiro, F. (2001). Eye movement sensitization and reprocessing: Basic principles, protocols, and procedures (2nd ed.). New York, NY: Guilford Press.

Shaw, R. (2004). The embodied psychotherapist: An exploration of the therapist's somatic phenomena within the therapeutic encounter. *Psychotherapy Research, 14*(3), 271–288.

Shepherd, G. M. (1983). *Neurobiology.* New York, NY: Oxford University Press.

Sherer, Y., Gerli, R., Vaudo, G., Schillaci, G., Gilburd, B., Giordano, A., . . . Sheonfeld, Y. (2005). Prevalence of antiphospholoid and antioxidized low-density lipoprotein antibodies in rheumatoid arthritis. *Annals of the New York Academy of Sciences, 1051,* 299–303.

Sherrington, C. (1906). *The integrative action of the nervous system.* London, England: Cambridge University Press.

Shewmon, D. A., Holmes, G. L., & Byrne, P. A. (1999). Consciousness in congenitally decorticate children: Developmental vegetative state as self-fulfilling prophecy. *Developmental Medicine and Child Neurology, 41,* 364–74.

Siegel, D. J. (1999). *The developing mind: Toward a neurobiology of interpersonal experience.* New York, NY: The Guilford Press.

Simons, S. H. P., van Dijk, M., Anand, K. J. S., Roofthooft, D., van Lingen, R. A., & Tibboel, D. (2003). Do we still hurt newborn babies? A prospective study of procedural pain and analgesia in neonates. *Archives of Pediatrics and Adolescent Medicine, 157,* 1058–64.

Singer, W. (1993). Synchronization of cortical activity and its putative role in information processing and learning. *Annual Review of Physiology, 55,* 349–374.

Singer, W. (2001). Consciousness and the binding problem. *Annals of the New York Academy of Sciences, 929,* 123–146.

Singer, W., Engel, A. K, Kreiter, A. K., Munk, M. H. J., Neuenschwander, S., & Roelfsema, P. R. (1997). Neuronal assemblies: Necessity, signature and detectability. *Trends in Cognitive Science, 1*(7), 252–261.

Sirven, J. L., & Glaser, D. S. (1998). Psychogenic nonepileptic seizures. Theoretic and clinical considerations. *Neuropsychiatry, Neuropsychology, and Behavioral Science, 27,* 225–235.

Slotnick, S. D. (2004). Visual memory and visual perception recruit common neural substrates. *Behavioral and Cognitive Neuroscience Reviews, 3*(4), 207–221.

Spitz, R. A. (1965). *The first year of life: A psychoanalytic study of normal and deviant development of object relations.* New York, NY: International Universities Press.

Squire, L. R., & Kandel, E. R. (1999). *Memory: From mind to molecules.* New York, NY: Scientific American Library.

Stallard, P., Williams, L., Lenton, S., & Velleman, R. (2001). Pain in cognitively impaired, non-communicating children. *Archives of Disease in Childhood, 85*(6), 460–462.

Steele, K., van der Hart, O., & Nijenhuis, E. R. S. (2001). Dependency in the treatment of complex posttraumatic stress disorder and dissociative disorders. *Journal of Trauma Dissociation, 2*(4), 79–116.

Steriade, M., Amzica, F., & Contreras, D. (1996). Synchronization of fast (30–40 Hz) spontaneous cortical rhythms during brain activtion. *Journal of Neuroscience, 16,* 392–417.

Steriade, M., CurroDossi, R., & Contreras, F. (1993). Electrophysiological properties of intralaminar thalamo–cortical cells discharging rhythmic 40 Hz spite bursts at 1000 Hz during waking and rapid eye movement sleep. *Neuroscience, 56,* 1–9.

Steriade, M., Jones, E. G., & Llinas, R. R. (1990). *Thalamic oscillations and signaling.* New York: Wiley.

Stern, D. (1985). *The interpersonal world of the infant: A view from psychoanalysis and developmental psychology.* New York, NY: Basic Books.

Stickgold, R. (2002). EMDR: A putative neurobiological mechanism of action. *Journal of Clinical Psychology, 58*(1), 61–75.

Stickgold, R. (2005). Sleep-dependent memory consolidation. *Nature, 437,* 1272–1278.

Stickgold, R. (2007). Of sleep, memories and trauma. *Nature Neuroscience, 10*(5), 540–542.

Stickgold, R. (2008). Sleep dependent memory processing and EMDR action. *Journal of EMDR Practice and Research, 2*(4), 289–299.

Stickgold, R., Scott, L., Rittenhouse, C., & Hobson, J. A. (1999). Sleep induced changes in associative memory. *Journal of Cognitive Neuroscience, 11,* 182–193.

Sullivan, H. S. (1940). *Conceptions of modern psychiatry.* New York, NY: Norton.

Szelenyi, J., & Vizi, E. S. (2007). The Catecholamine–cytokine balance: Interaction between the brain and the immune system. *Annals of New York Academy of Sciences, 1113,* 311–324.

Teicher, M. H., Glod, C. A., Surrey, J., & Swett, C. (1993). Early childhood abuse and limbic system ratings in adult psychiatric outpatients. *The Journal of Neuropsychiatry and Clinical Neurosciences, 5*(3), 301–306.

Terr, L. C. (1988). What happens to early memories of trauma? A study of twenty children under age at the time of documented traumatic events. *Journal of the American Academy of Child and Adolescent Psychiatry, 27,* 96–104.

Thayer, J. F., & Lane, R. D. (2009). Claude Bernard and the heart–brain connection: Further elaboration of a model of neurovisceral integration. *Neuroscience and Biobehavioral Review, 33,* 81–88.

Thompson, M. E., & Barkhuizen, A. (2003). Fibromyalgia, hepatitis C infection, and the cytokine connection. *Current Pain & Headache Reports, 7,* 342–347.

Thompson, R. F., & Spencer, W. A. (1966). Habituation: A model phenomenon for the study of the neural substrates of behavior. *Psychological Review, 173,* 16–43.

Tigh, T. J., & Leaton, R. N. (1976). *Habituation: Perspectives from child development, animal behavior and neurophysiology.* Hillsdale, NJ: Erlbaum.

Tronick, E. Z., & Weinberg, M. K. (1997). Depressed mothers and infants: Failure to form dyadic states of consciousness. In L. Murray & P. J. Cooper (Eds.), *Postpartum depression in child development* (pp. 54–81). New York, NY: Guilford.

Tucker, D. M. (1992). Developing emotions and cortical networks. In M. R. Gunar & C. A. Nelson (Eds.), *Minnesota Symposium on Child Psychology, 24, Developmental Behavioral Neurosciences* (pp. 75–128). Hillside, NJ: Laurence Erlbaum Associates.

Tucker, D. M., Luu, P., & Pribram, K. H. (1995). Social and emotional self-regulation. *Annals of the New York Academy of Sciences, 769,* 213–239.

Tulving, E. (1972). Episodic and semantic memory. In E. Tulving & W. Donaldson (eds). Organization of memory, (pp. 381–403). New York: Academic Press.

Turk, D. J., Heatherton, T., Kelley, W. M., Funnell, M. G., Gazzaniga, M. S., & Macrae, C. N. (2002). Mike or me? Self-recognition in a split-brain patient. *Nature Neuroscience, 5*(9), 841–842.

Turk, D. J., Heatherton, T. F., Macrae, C. N., Kelley, W. M., & Gazzaniga, M. S. (2003). Out of contact, out of mind: The distributed nature of the self. *Annals of the New York Academy of Sciences, 1001,* 65–78.

Vaadia, E., Haalman, I., Abeles, M., Bergman, H., Prut, Y., Slovin, H., & Aertsen, A. (1995). Dynamics of neuronal interactions in monkey cortex in relation to behavioural events. *Nature, 373,* 515–518.

Van der Hart, O., & Nijenhuis, E. R. S. (1998). Recovered memories of abuse and dissociative identity disorder. *British Journal Psychiatry, 173,* 537–538.

Van der Hart, O., Nijenhuis, E. R. S., & Steele, J. (2005). Dissociation: An insufficiently recognize major feature of complex posttraumatic stress disorder. *Journal of Traumatic Stress, 18,* 413–424.

Van der Hart, O., Nijenhuis, E. R. S., & Steele, K. (2006). *The haunted self: Structural dissociation in the treatment of chronic traumatization.* New York, NY: W. W. Norton & Co.

Van der Hart, O., Nijenhuis, E. R. S., Steele, K., & Brown, D. (2004). Trauma related dissociation: conceptual clarity lost and found. *Australian and New Zealand Journal Psychiatry, 38,* 906–914.

Van der Hart, O., van der Kolk, B. A., & Boon, S. (1996). The treatment of dissociative disorders. In J. D. Bremner and C. R. Marmar (Eds.), *Trauma memory and dissociation.* Washington, DC: American Psychiatric Press.

Van der Kolk, B. A. (1994). The body keeps the score: Memory and the evolving psychobiology of PTSD. *Harvard Review of Psychiatry, 1,* 253–265.

Van der Kolk, B. A. (1996a). The body keeps the score: Approaches to the psychobiology of posttraumatic stress disorder. In B. A. van der Kolk, A. C. McFarlane, & L. Weisaeth (Eds.), *Traumatic stress: The effects of overwhelming experience on mind, body and society* (pp. 214–241). New York, NY: The Guilford Press.

Van der Kolk, B. A. (1996b). The complexity of adaptation to trauma: Self regulation, stimulus discrimination, and character development. In B. A. van der Kolk, A. C. McFarlane, & L. Weisaeth (Eds.). *Traumatic stress: The effects of overwhelming experience on mind, body and society* (pp. 182–213). New York, NY: The Guilford Press.

Van der Kolk, B. A. (2001). The assessment and treatment of complex PTSD. In R. Yehuda (Ed.), *Traumatic stress*. New York, NY: American Psychiatric Press.

Van der Kolk, B. A. (2005). Developmental trauma disorder: Toward a rational diagnosis for children with complex trauma histories. *Psychiatric Annals, 35*, 401–408.

Van der Kolk, B. A. (2006). Clinical implications of neuroscience research in PTSD. *Annals of the New York Academy of Sciences, 1071*, 277–293.

Van der Kolk, B. A., & d'Andrea, W. (2010). Toward a developmental trauma disorder diagnosis for childhood interpersonal trauma. In R. A. Lanius, E. Vermetten, & C. Pain (Eds.), *The impact of early life trauma on health and disease: The hidden epidemic* (pp. 57–68). New York, NY: Cambridge University Press.

Van der Kolk, B. A., & McFarlane, A. C. (1996). The black hole of trauma. In B. A. van der Kolk, A. C. McFarlane, & L. Weisaeth (Eds.). *Traumatic stress: The effects of overwhelming experience on mind, body and society* (pp. 3–23). New York, NY: The Guilford Press.

Van der Kolk, B. A., Perry, C., & Herman, J. L. (1991). Childhood origins of self-destructive behavior. *American Journal of Psychiatry, 148*, 1665–1671.

Van der Kolk, B., & van der Hart, O. (1989). The intrusive past: The flexibility of memory and the engraving of trauma. *American Imago, 48*, 425–454.

Van der Kolk, B. A., van der Hart, O., & Marmar, C. R. (1996). Dissociation and information processing in posttraumatic stress disorder. In B. A. van der Kolk, A. C. McFarlane, & L. Weisaeth (Eds.). *Traumatic stress: The effects of overwhelming experience on mind, body and society* (pp. 303–330). New York, NY: The Guilford Press.

Van der Kolk, B. A., Weisaeth, L., & Van der Hart, O. (1996). History of trauma in psychiatry. In B. A. van der Kolk, A. C. McFarlane, & L. Weisaeth (Eds.). *Traumatic stress: The effects of overwhelming experience on mind, body and society* (pp. 47–74). New York, NY: The Guilford Press.

Von der Malsburg, C. (1973). Self organizing of orientation in sensitive cells in the striated cortex. *Kybernetic, 14*, 85–100.

Wagner, U., Gais, S., Haider, H., Verleger, R., & Born, J. (2004). Sleep inspires insight. *Nature, 427*(6972), 352–355.

Wang, P. W., Chen, I. Y., Liu, R. T., Hsieh, C. J., His, E., & Juo, S. H. (2007). Cytotoxic T lymphocyte-associated molecule-4 gene polymorphism and hyperthyroid Graves' disease relapse after antithyroid drug withdrawal: A follow-up study. *Journal of Clinical Endocrinological Metabolism, 92*(7), 2513–2518.

Wang, W., Dow, K. E., & Fraser, D. D. (2001). Elevated corticotrophin-release hormone/corticotrophin-releasing hormone-R1 expression in postmortem brain obtained from children with generalized epilepsy. *Annals of Neurology, 50*, 404–409.

Watkins, H. H. (1978). Ego states therapy. In J. G. Watkins (Ed.), *The therapeutic self* (pp. 360–398). New York, NY: Human Sciences Press.

Watkins, J. G. (1949). *Hypnotherapy of war neuroses*. New York, NY: Ronald Press.

Watkins, J. G. (1977). The psychodynamic manipulation of ego states in hypnotherapy. In F. Antonelli (Ed.), *Therapy in psychosomatic medicine, 2,* 389–403.

Watkins, J. G., & Johnson, R. (1982). *We, the divided self.* New York, NY: Irvington.

Watkins, J. G., & Watkins, H. H. (1997). *Ego states: Theory and therapy.* New York: Norton.

Watkins, L. R., & Maier, S. F. (2000). The pain of being sick: Implications of immune-to-brain communication for understanding pain. *Annual Review of Psychology, 51,* 29–57.

Watkins, L. R., & Maier, S. F. (2005). Immune regulation of central nervous system functions: From sickness responses to pathological pain. *Journal of Internal Medicine, 257*(2), 139–55.

Whittling, W., & Schweiger, E. (1993). Neuroendocrine brain asymmetry and physical complaints. *Neuropsychologia, 31,* 591–608.

Williams, R. W., & Herrup, K. (1988). The control of neuron number. *Annual Review of Neuroscience, 11,* 423–453.

Willshaw, D. J. (1981). Holography, associative memory, and inductive generalization. In G. E. Hinton & J. A. Anderson (Eds.), *Parallel models of associative memory* (pp. 83–104). Hillsdale, NJ: Erlbaum.

Wilson, M. A., & McNaughton, B. L. (1994). Reactivation of hippocampal ensemble memories during sleep. *Science, 265,* 676–679.

Winnicott, D. W. (1956). Primary maternal preoccupation. In *Through paediatrics to psycho-analysis* (pp. 300–305). New York, NY: Basic Books.

Winnicott, D. W. (1965). Ego distortion in terms of true and false self. In *The maturational processes and the facilitating environment* (pp. 37–55). New York, NY: International Universities Press.

Winson, J. (1985). *Brain and psyche: The biology of the unconscious.* New York, NY: Doubleday/Anchor Press.

Witte, T. (2005). Antifodrin antibodies in Sjögren's syndrome: A review. *Annals of the New York Academy of Sciences, 1051,* 235–239.

Wolff, P. (1987). *The development of behavioral states and the expression of emotion in early infancy.* Chicago, IL: University of Chicago Press.

Yanus, M. B. (2007). Role of central sensitization in symptoms beyond muscle pain, and the evaluation of a patient with widespread pain. *Best Practice & Research Clinical Rheumatology, 21*(3), 481–497.

Yehuda, R. (1997). Sensitization of the hypothalamic–pituitary–adrenal axis in post-traumatic stress disorder. *Annals of the New York Academy of Sciences, 821,* 57–82.

Yehuda, R. (2002). Current status of cortisol findings in posttraumatic stress disorder. *Psychiatric Clinics of North America* (review), *25,* 341–368.

Yehuda, R. (2006). Advances in understanding neuroendocrine alterations in PTSD and their therapeutic implications. *Annals of the New York Academy of Sciences, 1071,* 137–166.

Yehuda, R., Engel, S. M., Brand, S. R., Seckl, J., Marcus, S. M., & Berkowitz, G. S. (2005). Transgenerational effects of posttraumatic stress disorder in babies of mothers exposed to the World Trade Center attacks during pregnancy. *Journal of Clinical Endocrinology & Metabolism, 90,* 4115–4118.

Yehuda, R., Teicher, M. H., Seckl, J. R., Grossman, R. A., Morris, A., & Bierer, L. M. (2007). Parental posttraumatic stress disorder as a vulnerability factor for low cortisol trait in offspring of holocaust survivors. *Archives of General Psychiatry, 64*(9), 1040–1048.

Yoshida, M., Yokoo, H., Tanaka, T., Mizoguchi, K., Emoto, H., Ishii, H., & Tanaka, M. (1993). Facilitory modulation of mesolimbic dopamine neuronal activity by m-opioid agonist and nicotine as examined with *in vivo* microdialysis. *Brain Research, 624,* 277–280.

Zagon, I. S., McLaughlin, P. J., & Smith, S. (1977). Neural populations in the human cerebellum: Estimations from isolated cell nuclei. *Brain Research, 127,* 279–282.

Zald, D. H., & Kim, S. W. (1996). Anatomy and function of the orbital frontal cortex: Function and relevance to obsessive compulsive disorder. *Journal of Neuropsychiatry, 8,* 249–261.

Index